ESSENTIALS OF

HUMAN EMBRYOLOGY

ESSENTIALS OF

HUMAN EMBRYOLOGY

KEITH L. MOORE, Ph.D., F.I.A.C.

Professor of Anatomy and
Associate Dean, Basic Sciences
Faculty of Medicine
University of Toronto
Toronto, Ontario, Canada

Formerly Head of Anatomy
University of Manitoba
and later Chairman of Anatomy
University of Toronto

Illustrated by

MARLENE HERBST, B.A., B.Sc., AAM
MEGAN THOMPSON, B.A., B.Sc., AAM

1988   B.C. Decker Inc • Toronto • Philadelphia

Publisher

B.C. Decker Inc
3228 South Service Road
Burlington, Ontario   L7N 3H8

B.C. Decker Inc
320 Walnut Street
Suite 400
Philadelphia, Pennsylvania   19106

Sales and Distribution

United States and Possessions	**The C.V. Mosby Company** 11830 Westline Industrial Drive Saint Louis, Missouri 63146
Canada	**The C.V. Mosby Company, Ltd.** 5240 Finch Avenue East, Unit No. 1 Scarborough, Ontario M1S 5P2
United Kingdom, Europe and the Middle East	**Blackwell Scientific Publications, Ltd.** Osney Mead, Oxford OX2 OEL, England
Australia and New Zealand	**Harcourt Brace Jovanovich Group (Australia) Pty Limited** 30–52 Smidmore Street Marrickville, N.S.W. 2204 Australia
Japan	**Igaku-Shoin Ltd.** Tokyo International P.O. Box 5063 1–28–36 Hongo, Bunkyo-ku, Tokyo 113, Japan
Asia	**Info-Med Ltd.** 802–3 Ruttonjee House 11 Duddell Street Central Hong Kong
South Africa	**Libriger Book Distributors** Warehouse Number 8 ''Die Ou Looiery'' Tannery Road Hamilton, Bloemfontein 9300
South America	**Inter-Book Marketing Services** Rua das Palmeriras, 32 Apto. 701 222–70 Rio de Janeiro RJ, Brazil

Essentials of Human Embryology

ISBN 0-941158-97-7

Library of Congress catalog card number: 87–72965   Printed in Hong Kong

10 9 8 7 6 5 4 3 2 1

To our daughter
Laurel Ann
in celebration of her recent graduation
from the University of Manitoba

PREFACE

Essentials of Human Embryology is intended not only as an overview for beginning students, but also as a quick review for students who have taken courses in human embryology and who are preparing for the National Board Examinations (NBME) or for other comprehensive examinations. It can be used in conjunction with the author's *Study Guide and Review Manual of Human Embryology*, which contains National Board format questions. This little book would also help residents prepare for their specialty examinations and aid medical practitioners who wish to refresh their knowledge of human development.

The book is copiously illustrated in color because most developmental processes can be visualized and understood with minimal text, that is if they are shown diagrammatically. The notes are intended to emphasize important points and to explain difficult stages of development, both normal and abnormal.

Essentials of Human Embryology provides a visual summary of human development and an outline of its most important concepts. The confrontation of text and illustrations aids both the visualization of normal human development and the understanding of the causes of common congenital malformations (birth defects).

As with my other textbooks, *The Developing Human: Clinically Oriented Embryology* and *Before We Are Born: Basic Embryology and Birth Defects*, this new book derives from my 32 years of teaching embryology to health sciences students.

During the preparation of this book, I have had the friendly assistance of several talented persons: Marlene Herbst and Megan Thompson who prepared all the illustrations and Karen McMurray who typed and proofread the manuscript. My wife and colleague, Marion, read and discussed the proofs with me. I also wish to thank Professor Harry Peery, who edited the copy. Most especially, thanks are due to Mr. Walter Bailey, President of B.C. Decker Inc., who took a special interest in this book and who was most helpful durings its preparation.

Keith L. Moore

CONTENTS

FIRST WEEK OF HUMAN DEVELOPMENT

FIRST WEEK OF HUMAN DEVELOPMENT

Human development begins after the union of male and female gametes or germ cells during a process known as **fertilization** (conception).

Fertilization is a sequence of events (Fig. 1–1) that begins with the contact of a **sperm** (spermatozoon) with a **secondary oocyte** (ovum) and ends with the fusion of their *pronuclei* (the haploid nuclei of the sperm and ovum) and the mingling of their chromosomes to form a new cell (see Fig. 1–1D). This fertilized ovum, known as a **zygote** (see Fig. 1–1E), is a large diploid cell that is the beginning, or *primordium, of a human being.*

Some 300 to 500 million sperms are deposited by a male who ejaculates into the vagina of a female during sexual intercourse. The sperms pass through the cervical canal, the uterine cavity, and along the uterine tube to its widest portion, known as the **ampulla**. The sperms retain their fertilizing power for two to three days.

Fertilization normally occurs in the ampulla of the uterine tube 12 to 24 hours after ovulation (see Fig. 1–1). As sperms approach the secondary oocyte, perforations develop in their acrosomes. During this process, known as the **acrosome reaction**, enzymes are released (see Fig. 1–1A). *Hyaluronidase* causes separation and sloughing of the corona radiata cells surrounding the ovum. *Acrosin* and *neuraminidase* facilitate the passage of a sperm through the zona pellucida, a rather thick amorphous membrane that surrounds the secondary oocyte. As soon as a sperm contacts the plasma membrane of the secondary oocyte, changes occur in the zona pellucida, known as the **zona reaction**; these changes normally prevent additional sperms from entering the secondary oocyte.

Sperm contact also induces the secondary oocyte to complete its second meiotic division, which forms a **mature ovum** and a second polar body. The nucleus of the ovum is known as the *female pronucleus.*

Once within the ovum's cytoplasm, the tail of the sperm degenerates, and its head enlarges to form the *male pronucleus* (see Fig. 1–1C). The male and female pronuclei approach each other and fuse (see Fig. 1–1D). The maternal and paternal chromosomes intermingle and a new diploid cell, the zygote, forms (see Fig. 1–1E).

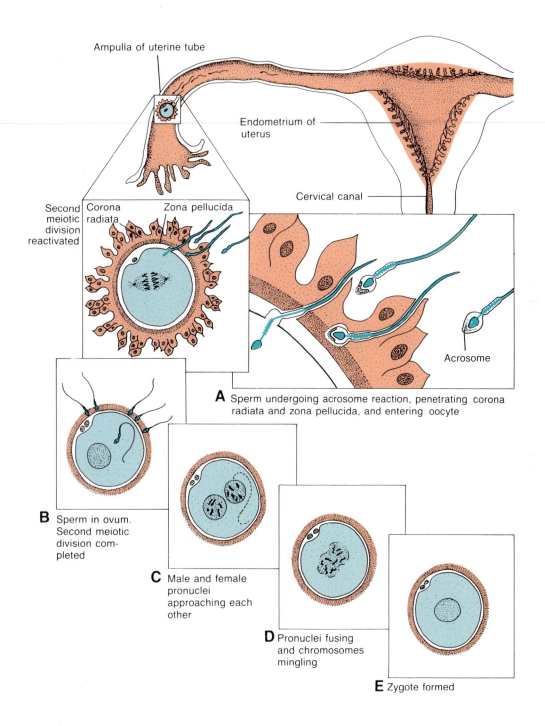

Figure 1–1 The mechanism of fertilization. The sequence of events begins with contact between a sperm and a secondary oocyte in the ampulla of the uterine tube and ends with formation of a zygote.

The **results of fertilization** are as follows:

1. *Restoration of the diploid number* (46) of chromosomes;
2. *Determination of the chromosomal sex of the embryo;*
3. *Variation of the human species* (owing to the new combination of chromosomes); and
4. *Initiation of cleavage* (mitotic division of the zygote into blastomeres).

As the zygote passes along the uterine tube to the uterus, it undergoes **cleavage**, which is a series of rapid *mitotic cell divisions* (Fig. 1–2). The new cells, known as **blastomeres**, become smaller with each division. After several divisions, a mulberry-shaped mass of 16 blastomeres forms. It is known as a **morula** (see Fig. 1–2D). This mass is still surrounded by the protective layer known as the *zona pellucida*. The morula forms as the developing human is about to enter the uterine cavity.

As soon as the morula enters the uterus, fluid begins to pass through the zona pellucida into the intercellular spaces between the blastomeres. Gradually these spaces become confluent and form a large cavity known as the **blastocyst cavity** (see Fig. 1–2E). As soon as this cavity is recognizable (about 4 days after fertilization), the developing embryo becomes known as a **blastocyst**.

As the amount of fluid in the blastocyst cavity increases, the cells become separated into two parts (see Fig. 1–2E) comprising (1) a flattened outer cell layer ("mass"), known as the **trophoblast**, which eventually gives rise to the embryonic part of the placenta, and (2) a group of centrally located cells known as the **inner cell mass** or embryoblast that is the primordium of the embryo.

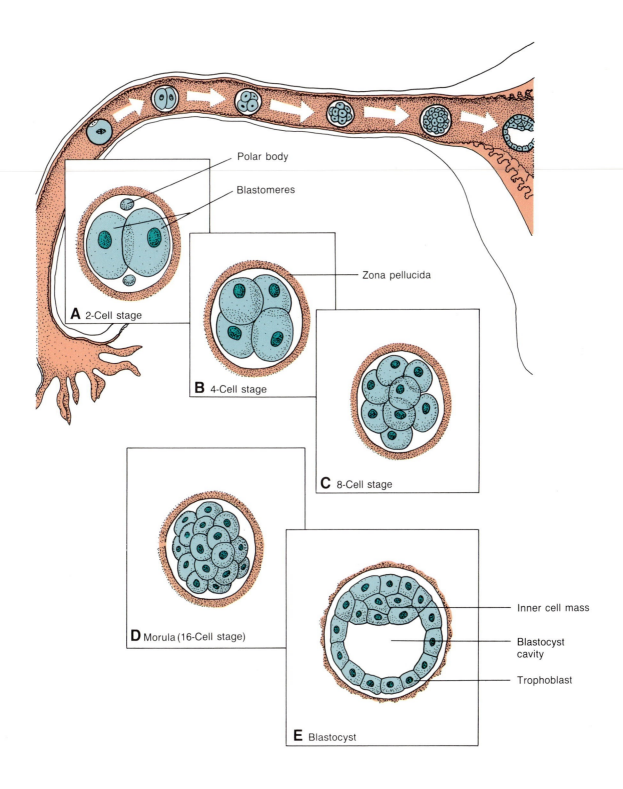

Polar body

Blastomeres

Zona pellucida

A 2-Cell stage

B 4-Cell stage

C 8-Cell stage

D Morula (16-Cell stage)

Inner cell mass

Blastocyst cavity

Trophoblast

E Blastocyst

Figure 1-2 Cleavage of the zygote and formation of the blastocyst. These initial stages of human development (1 to 4 days) occur in the uterine tube and after the uterus is entered. The blastocyst, a hollow ball of cells, has been sectioned to illustrate its internal structure.

The zona pellucida degenerates and disappears about 5 days after fertilization, and the blastocyst enlarges. The trophoblast attaches to the endometrial epithelium about six days after fertilization (see Fig. 1–3A). This begins the process known as **implantation**. The attached region of the trophoblast immediately differentiates into two layers, an internal *cellular layer* known as the **cytotrophoblast**, and an external *syncytial layer* known as the **syncytiotrophoblast** (see Fig. 1–3B). The latter is formed in the following manner. During this differentiation, cells in the cytotrophoblast layer divide and some migrate to the external layer where they fuse and lose their cell membranes. This produces the **multinucleate mass** or **syncytium** called the syncytiotrophoblast.

By the end of the first week, a layer of cuboidal cells, known as the **hypoblast** (primitive endoderm), forms on the ventral surface of the inner cell mass (see Fig. 1–3B), thereby forming the roof of the blastocyst cavity. The remaining cells of the inner cell mass give rise to the **epiblast** during the second week.

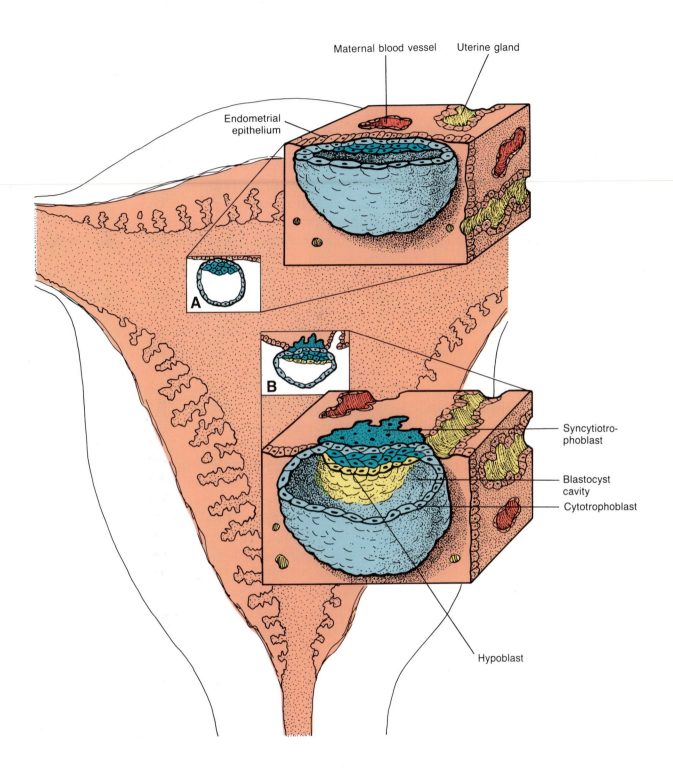

Figure 1-3 The early stages of implantation of the blastocyst into the endometrium on the posterior wall of the uterus. *A*, at six days the trophoblast is attached to the endometrial epithelium adjacent to the inner cell mass. *B*, at seven days the trophoblast has differentiated into two layers: syncytiotrophoblast and cytotrophoblast. The syncytiotrophoblast has started to invade the endometrium. A layer of cells, known as the hypoblast, has also formed on the ventral surface of the inner cell mass.

SUMMARY

Fertilization normally occurs in the ampulla of the uterine tube, not later than 24 hours after ovulation (see Fig. 1–1).

Fusion of the haploid *pronuclei* of the sperm and ovum converts the fertilized ovum into a **zygote**, a diploid cell (see Fig. 1–1E). The *chromosomal* or *primary sex of the embryo is established* at this time.

Cleavage of the zygote into blastomeres (smaller cells) occurs as the zygote passes along the uterine tube to the uterus (see Fig. 1–2). At the 12- to 16-cell stage, the developing human is called a **morula** (see Fig. 1–2D).

About **three days** after fertilization, the morula enters the uterus. Uterine fluid passes through the zona pellucida surrounding the morula. This fluid fills the spaces which appear between the central cells of the morula. These spaces soon coalesce to form a **blastocyst cavity** and, thus, the developing human is now called a **blastocyst** (see Fig. 1–2E).

The blastocyst forms **four to five days** after fertilization. The external cells of the blastocyst form a layer known as the **trophoblast** (see Fig. 1–2E). Subsequently, the trophoblast contributes to the formation of the embryonic part of the placenta. The internal cells of the blastocyst form a group known as the **inner cell mass.** As these cells are those which give rise to the embryo, they are often collectively called the **embryoblast.**

About **five days** after fertilization the zona pellucida disappears and the blastocyst enlarges. By the **sixth day**, the trophoblast attaches to the endometrial epithelium (see Fig. 1–3A). The attached region of the trophoblast, usually adjacent to the inner cell mass, differentiates into two layers (see Fig. 1–3B). The internal cellular layer, called the **cytotrophoblast**, gives rise to an external syncytial layer, called the **syncytiotrophoblast**. The syncytiotrophoblast invades the endometrial epithelium and connective tissue by the end of the **seventh day**. This erosion of maternal tissues is *the beginning of the implantation of the blastocyst.*

By the end of the first week, a layer of cells known as the **hypoblast** has formed on the ventral surface of the inner cell mass. It gives rise to the primitive endoderm. The remaining cells of the inner cell mass eventually form the **epiblast**.

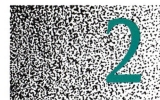

SECOND WEEK OF HUMAN DEVELOPMENT

SECOND WEEK OF HUMAN DEVELOPMENT

The second week of embryonic development is *characterized by the completion of implantation of the blastocyst* and further development of the trophoblast (Fig. 2–1). As implantation occurs, changes occur in the inner cell mass that produce a **bilaminar embryonic disc.** It is composed of two distinct layers: the *epiblast* and *hypoblast*; the *amniotic cavity and yolk sac develop* in association with these layers (see Fig. 2–1A and B).

As the blastocyst embeds itself in the endometrium of the uterus, more and more of its trophoblast comes into contact with the endometrial tissues. As a result, differentiation of the trophoblast continues until the wall of the blastocyst is composed of two complete layers of *cytotrophoblast* and *syncytiotrophoblast* (see Fig. 2–1C). As the syncytiotrophoblast layer expands, **lacunae** (small spaces) develop that soon become filled with maternal blood, cellular debris, and glandular secretions (see Fig. 2–1B). This material provides nutrition for the embryo. The lacunae gradually fuse to form **lacunar networks** (see Fig. 2–1C). As the syncytiotrophoblast erodes endometrial blood vessels, maternal blood flows in and out of the lacunar networks, establishing a **primitive uteroplacental circulation.** The developing embryo receives oxygen and nutrients from the maternal blood and disposes of its carbon dioxide and waste products into the mother's blood.

By *the tenth day after fertilization, the blastocyst is completely embedded in the endometrium* (see Fig. 2–1B), but is confined to its superficial compact layer. The implanted blastocyst produces a small elevated area of endometrium in which a **closing plug** of fibrin is visible for a day or two.

At the beginning of the second week, a small cavity appears between the inner cell mass and the two layers of the trophoblast. This space is the beginning of the **amniotic cavity** (see Fig. 2–1A). Concurrently, morphologic changes occur in the inner cell mass that result in the formation of a flat, essentially circular plate composed of two layers (see Fig. 2–1B). This bilaminar area, called the **embryonic disc**, consists of two layers: (1) the *epiblast*, consisting of high columnar cells related to the amniotic cavity; and (2) the *hypoblast*, consisting of cuboidal cells adjacent to the blastocyst cavity, now known as the *primary yolk sac.*

As the amniotic cavity enlarges, it acquires a thin, epithelial domed roof called the **amnion** (see Fig. 2–1B and C). The cells that form the amnion, called *amnioblasts*, arise from the cytotrophoblast. The embryonic epiblast forms the floor of the amniotic cavity and is continuous with the amnion peripherally. As the amnion forms, other cells arise from the cytotrophoblast and form a thin *exocoelomic membrane* (see Fig. 2–1B). This membrane is continuous with the hypoblast of the embryonic disc and forms the wall of the **primary yolk sac.**

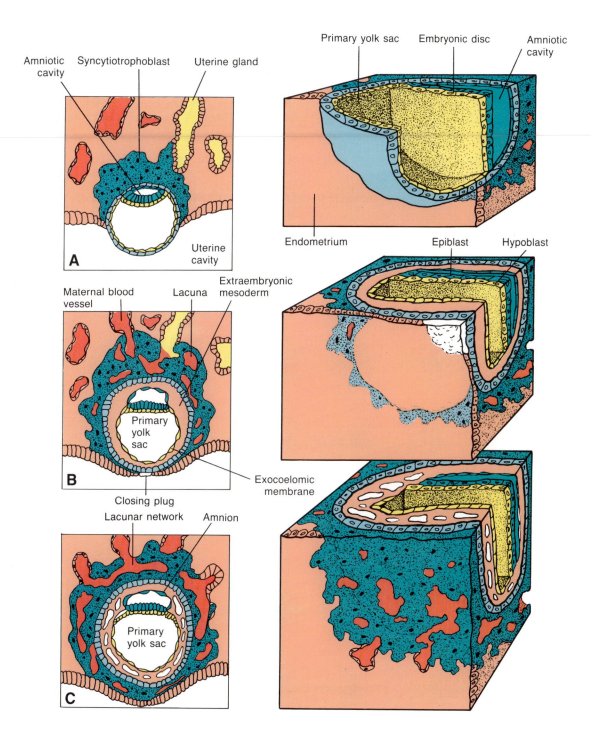

Figure 2–1 The final stages of implantation of the blastocyst. Formation of the amniotic cavity and primary yolk sac is also illustrated. A three-dimensional drawing is to the right of each section of the blastocyst. *A*, 8-day blastocyst partially implanted in the endometrium; *B*, 10-day blastocyst completely implanted in the endometrium; *C*, 12-day blastocyst showing the development of lacunar networks in the syncytiotrophoblast.

Further delamination of cytotrophoblastic cells gives rise to a thick layer of loosely-arranged cells called the **extraembryonic mesoderm** (see Fig. 2–1B). This layer completely fills the space between the trophoblast externally and the amnion and primary yolk sac internally.

By the middle of the second week, *isolated spaces appear in the extraembryonic mesoderm* (see Fig. 2–1C). These spaces soon coalesce to form a single large cavity called the **extraembryonic coelom** (see Fig. 2–2A). This coelomic cavity is also called the chorionic cavity when the **chorionic sac** forms at the end of the second week (see Fig. 2–2C). The wall of the chorionic sac is formed by the **chorion**, which is composed of a layer of extraembryonic mesoderm and the two layers of trophoblast.

By the end of the second week, **primary chorionic villi** have developed as outgrowths of the trophoblast from the chorion. They consist of a core of cytotrophoblast covered by a thick layer of syncytiotrophoblast (see Fig. 2–2C). These primary villi are the primordia of the chorionic villi of the **placenta**. By the end of the second week, a **prochordal plate** has developed as a localized thickening of hypoblast at the cranial end of the embryonic disc (see Fig. 2–2C). *The prochordal plate is an organizer of the head region* and indicates where the mouth of the embryo will develop.

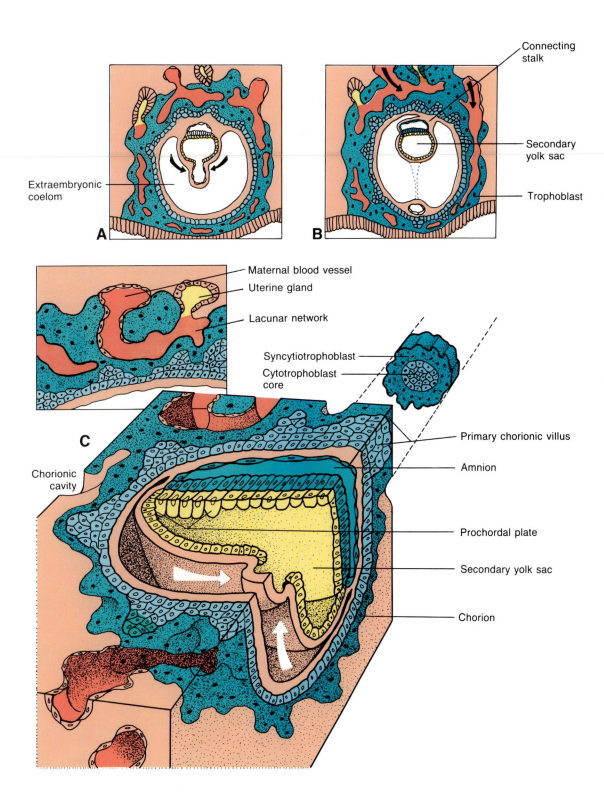

Figure 2–2 Sections of completely implanted blastocysts at the end of the second week, illustrating how the secondary yolk sac forms. The presence of primary chorionic villi on the wall of the chorionic sac is characteristic of blastocysts at the end of the second week. A primitive uteroplacental circulation is now present.

SUMMARY

The *amniotic cavity* develops between the epiblast and the cytotrophoblast (see Fig. 2–1A) and is soon enclosed by the **amnion** (see Fig. 2–1C). This epithelial layer is derived from the cytotrophoblast and is attached to the edges of the epiblast of the embryonic disc.

As implantation of the blastocyst occurs, two distinct embryonic layers, the *epiblast* and the *hypoblast*, differentiate from the inner cell mass. They constitute the **bilaminar embryonic disc** (see Fig. 2–1B).

The wall of the **primary yolk sac** develops from the exocoelomic membrane that is formed by cells that delaminate from the cytotrophoblast. The wall of the yolk sac is continuous with the hypoblast of the embryonic disc which forms its roof (see Fig. 2–1B).

Extraembryonic mesoderm also forms from cells that delaminate from the cytotrophoblast (see Fig. 2–1B). It completely fills the space between the amniotic and yolk sacs and the trophoblast. Spaces develop in the extraembryonic mesoderm (see Fig. 2–1C) which soon coalesce to form a large cavity known as the **extraembryonic coelom** (see Fig. 2–2A). This cavity splits the extraembryonic mesoderm into somatic and splanchnic layers and is called the chorionic cavity when the **chorionic sac** forms (see Fig. 2–2C).

The primitive yolk sac becomes reduced in size and is then known as the **secondary yolk sac** (see Fig. 2–2B). *The yolk sac contains no yolk* but is involved in the transfer of nutrients and oxygen to the embryo from the maternal blood. These substances diffuse through the **chorion**, enter the extraembryonic coelom, and pass along the wall of the yolk sac to the embryonic disc (primordium of the embryo).

By the end of the second week, the embryonic disc and its associated amniotic and yolk sacs are attached to the chorionic sac by a slender band of extraembryonic mesoderm known as the **connecting stalk** (see Fig. 2–2B). The connecting stalk is the primordium of the *umbilical cord*.

The implantation of the blastocyst is the prominent feature of the second week of development and may be summarized as follows (see Fig. 2–1):

1. The *syncytiotrophoblast erodes* the endometrial epithelium, stroma, blood vessels, and glands;
2. Lacunae (spaces) develop in the syncytiotrophoblast that soon coalesce to form **lacunar networks**;
3. Maternal blood seeps into and out of the lacunar networks, establishing a primitive *uteroplacental circulation*; and
4. The defect in the endometrial epithelium, through which the blastocyst passed, disappears by the end of the second week as the endometrial epithelium regenerates.

Implantation of the blastocyst normally occurs in the body of the uterus, usually in its anterior or posterior walls, but various extrauterine, or **ectopic, implantations** may occur. The most common location of ectopic gestations is in the uterine tube, but, in rare instances, implantations may occur in the ovary, peritoneal cavity, or cervix.

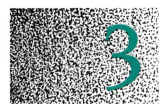

THIRD WEEK OF HUMAN DEVELOPMENT

THIRD WEEK OF HUMAN DEVELOPMENT

The third week is the beginning of a 6-week period of rapid development of the embryo from the embryonic disc that formed during the second week. *The third week of development of the embryo coincides with the week that follows the first missed menstrual period.*

GASTRULATION

Major changes occur in the developing embryo as the bilaminar embryonic disc is converted into a **trilaminar embryonic disc** composed of *three germ layers* (Fig. 3–1). The process of germ layer formation, called *gastrulation*, is the beginning of **embryogenesis** (formation of the embryo).

Gastrulation begins at the end of the first week with the appearance of the *hypoblast*; it continues during the second week with the formation of the *epiblast*; and is completed during the third week with the formation of intraembryonic mesoderm by the primitive streak (see Fig. 3–1). The **three primary germ layers** are called *ectoderm, mesoderm,* and *endoderm.* As the embryo develops, these layers give rise to the tissues and organs of the embryo.

The Primitive Streak

At the beginning of the third week, a thick *linear band of epiblast,* known as the primitive streak, appears caudally in the median plane of the dorsal aspect of the embryonic disc (see Fig. 3–1A). The primitive streak results from the accumulation or ''heaping up'' of cells of the epiblast as they proliferate and migrate to the center of the embryonic disc. As the primitive streak elongates by the addition of cells to its caudal end, cells at its cranial end proliferate to form an elevated **primitive knot** (see Figs. 3–1B and 3–2A).

The proliferation and migration of cells from the primitive streak give rise to *mesenchyme,* also called *mesoblast,* a loose embryonic connective tissue. Cells from the primitive streak spread laterally, cranially, and caudally. Some of these mesenchymal cells aggregate to form a layer between the epiblast and the hypoblast known as the embryonic mesoderm (see Figs. 3–1B and 3–2A). Some mesenchymal cells invade the hypoblast and displace most of its cells laterally. This newly-formed layer is known as the *embryonic endoderm.* The epiblastic cells that remain on the surface of the embryonic disc form the layer called the *embryonic ectoderm.*

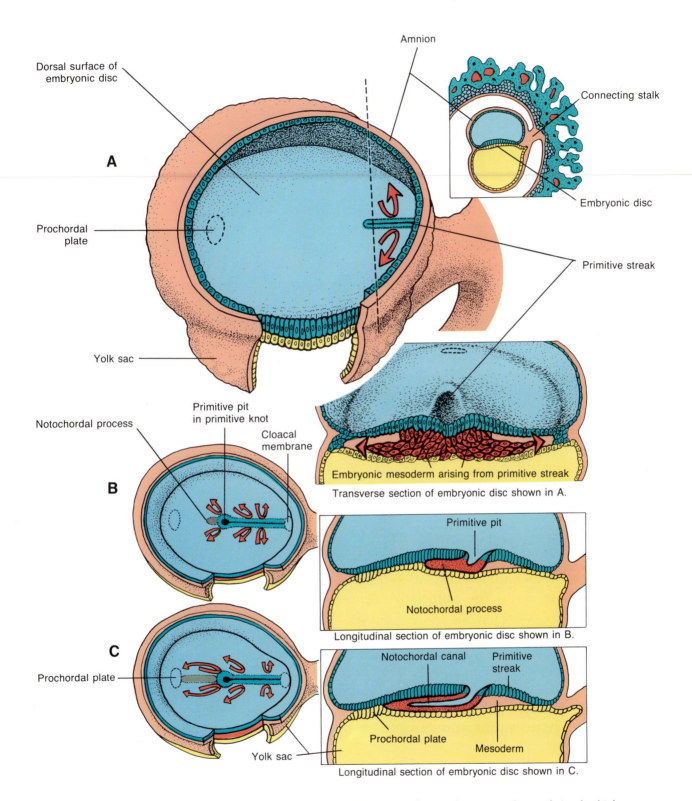

Figure 3–1 Schematic drawings of the embryonic disc and its associated extraembryonic membranes during the third week. *A*, the amniotic cavity has been opened to show the primitive streak, a midline thickening of the epiblast. Part of the yolk sac has also been cut away to show the bilaminar embryonic disc (epiblast and hypoblast). The transverse section (*lower right* of *A*) illustrates the proliferation and migration of mesenchymal cells from the primitive streak to form embryonic mesoderm. *B* and *C*, drawings illustrating early formation of the notochordal process from the primitive knot of the primitive streak. In the longitudinal sections on the right side, note that the notochordal process grows cranially in the median plane between the embryonic ectoderm (*blue*) and endoderm (*yellow*).

The embryonic ectoderm gives rise to the epidermis; the nervous system; the sensory epithelium of the eye, ear, and nose; and the enamel of the teeth. The embryonic endoderm forms the linings of the digestive and respiratory tracts. The embryonic mesoderm becomes muscle, connective tissue, bone, and blood vessels.

The Notochordal Process

From the primitive knot of the primitive streak, mesenchymal cells migrate cranially under the embryonic ectoderm in the median plane. These cells form a midline *cellular cord*, known as the notochordal process (see Fig. 3–1B) that grows cranially between embryonic ectoderm and endoderm until it reaches the **prochordal plate** (see Fig. 3–1C), the future site of the *mouth*. The notochordal process can extend no further because the prochordal plate, composed of endoderm, is firmly attached to the overlying ectoderm. The two layers that are fused in this area form the *oropharyngeal membrane* (see Fig. 3–2B).

Caudal to the primitive streak is a circular area known as the *cloacal membrane* (see Fig. 3–1B). Here the embryonic disc also remains bilaminar because the embryonic ectoderm and endoderm are fused. The cloacal membrane indicates the future site of the *anus*.

The primitive streak continues to form mesoderm until about the end of the fourth week. Thereafter it diminishes in relative size and becomes an insignificant structure in the sacrococcygeal region of the embryo. Normally, it degenerates and disappears but remnants of it may give rise to a tumor known as a *sacrococcygeal teratoma*.

The Notochord

The notochord is a cellular cord that *develops by transformation of the notochordal process* (Fig. 3–2). The notochord defines the primitive axis of the embryo and gives it some rigidity. During later development, the vertebral column forms around the notochord. By the end of the third week, the notochord is almost completely formed and extends from the oropharyngeal membrane cranially to the primitive knot caudally (Fig. 3–3).

The notochord degenerates and disappears during the fetal period in those locations where it is incorporated in the bodies of the vertebra. However, it persists between the vertebrae to form the *nucleus pulposus* of each intervertebral disc.

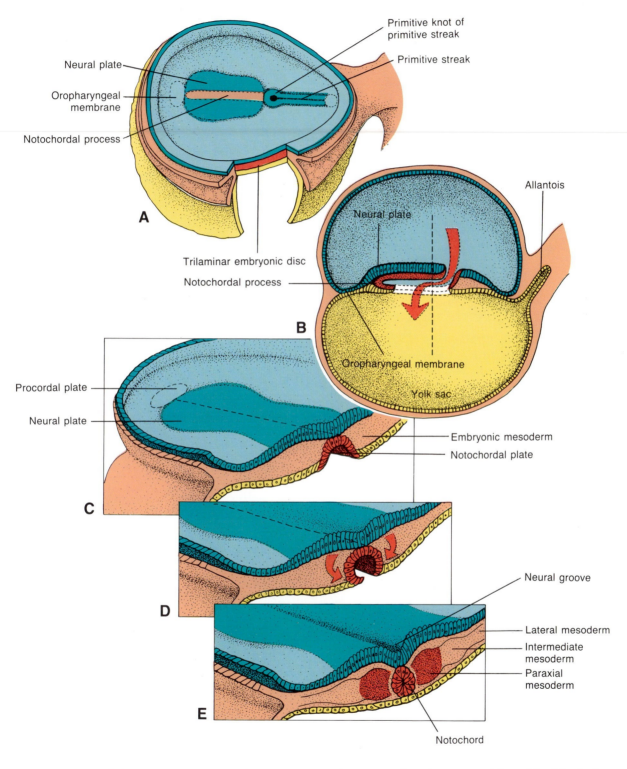

Figure 3–2 Schematic drawings of the embryonic disc and its associated membranes around the middle of the third week. *A*, the notochordal process and associated mesenchyme have induced the overlying ectoderm to form the neural plate. *B*, longitudinal section of the embryonic disc showing that the ventral wall of the notochordal process has degenerated. *C*, schematic transverse section of the embryonic disc at the level indicated in *B*, showing the notochordal plate. *D*, the arrows indicate infolding of the notochordal plate to form the notochord. *E*, the notochord has now formed, the endodermal layer is complete, and the embryonic mesoderm has differentiated into three regions.

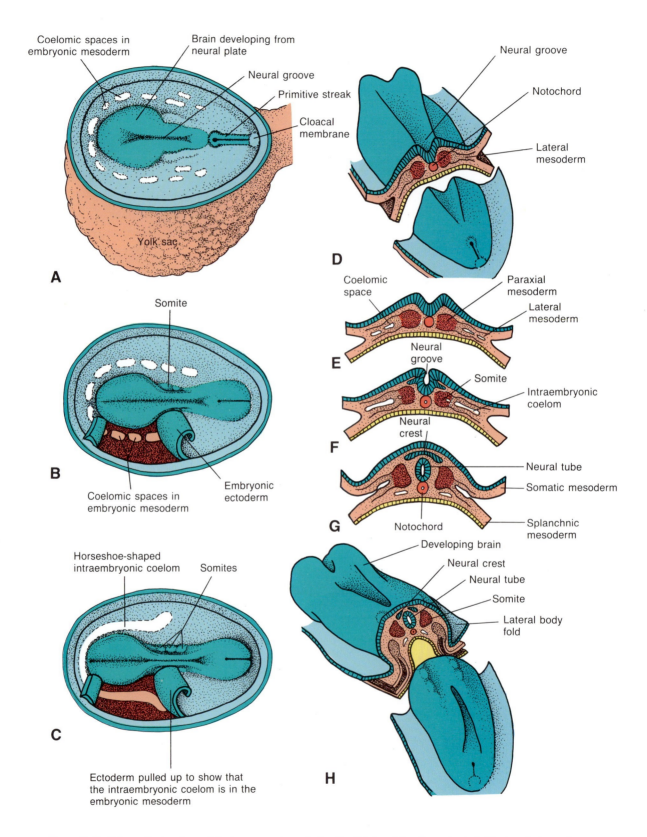

Figure 3–3 Schematic drawings of the human embryo during the third and fourth weeks. *Left side,* dorsal views of the developing embryo illustrating early formation of the brain, intraembryonic coelom, and somites. *Right side,* schematic transverse sections illustrating formation of the neural crest, neural tube, intraembryonic coelom, and somites.

NEURULATION

The process of formation of the *neural plate, neural folds,* and *neural tube* is called neurulation (see Figs. 3–2 and 3–3).

The Neural Plate

As the notochord develops, the embryonic ectoderm lying over both the notochord and the adjacent mesenchyme thickens to form the neural plate (see Fig. 3–2A and B). *It is the developing notochord and the mesenchyme adjacent to it that induce the overlying embryonic ectoderm to form the neural plate,* the primordium of the central nervous system (the brain and spinal cord).

The neural plate first appears near the primitive knot, but as the notochordal process elongates and the notochord forms, the neural plate enlarges and invaginates along its central axis to form a *neural groove,* which has *neural folds* on each side of it (see Figs. 3–2 and 3–3).

The Neural Tube

By the end of the third week, the *neural folds* have approached each other in the median plane and fused, converting the neural plate into a neural tube (see Fig. 3–3F and G). Formation of this tube begins near the middle of the embryo and progresses toward its cranial and caudal ends.

The Neural Crest

As the neural folds fuse to form the neural tube, some neuroectodermal cells, which lie along the crest of each fold, migrate ventrolaterally on each side of the neural tube (see Fig. 3–3G). Initially, these cells form an irregular elongated mass called the *neural crest,* located between the neural tube and the overlying surface ectoderm. The neural crest soon divides into right and left parts that migrate to the dorsolateral aspects of the neural tube (see Fig. 3–3H).

Neural crest cells migrate widely in the embryo and give rise to the *spinal ganglia* (dorsal root ganglia) and the ganglia of the autonomic nervous system. They also contribute to the ganglia of some cranial nerves and form the sheaths of peripheral nerves. Neural crest cells form the meninges (covering membranes) of the brain and spinal cord and give rise to pigment cells, the suprarenal medulla (adrenal medulla), and several skeletal and muscular components in the head.

DEVELOPMENT OF SOMITES

As the notochord and neural tube form, the adjacent mesoderm forms longitudinal columns called *paraxial mesoderm* (see Figs. 3–2E and 3–3E). These columns divide into paired cuboidal bodies called *somites* (see Fig. 3–3B and C). At the end of the third week, the first pair of somites develops a short distance caudal to the cranial end of the notochord. Subsequent pairs form in a craniocaudal sequence. During the *somite period of development* (days 20 to 30), the somites are used as one of the criteria for determining an embryo's age.

The somites form distinct surface elevations on the embryo and are somewhat triangular in transverse sections (see Fig. 3–3H). Mesenchymal cells from the somites give rise to most of the axial skeleton (vertebral column, ribs, sternum, and skull) and associated musculature, as well as to the adjacent dermis of the skin.

DEVELOPMENT OF INTRAEMBRYONIC COELOM

The intraembryonic coelom (primitive embryonic body cavity) first appears as *coelomic spaces* or cavities in the lateral mesoderm (see Fig. 3–3B and F), and in the mesoderm that will form the heart (*cardiogenic mesoderm*). These coelomic spaces soon coalesce to form a horseshoe-shaped cavity called the *intraembryonic coelom* (see Fig. 3–3C).

The intraembryonic coelom divides the lateral mesoderm into two layers, *a somatic or parietal layer* that is continuous with the extraembryonic mesoderm covering the amnion, and a *splanchnic or visceral layer* that is continuous with the extraembryonic mesoderm covering the yolk sac (see Fig. 3–3G). During the second month, the intraembryonic coelom is divided into three body cavities: (1) the *pericardial cavity* around the heart, (2) the *pleural cavities* around the lungs, and (3) the *peritoneal cavity* around the abdominal and pelvic organs.

THE PRIMITIVE CARDIOVASCULAR SYSTEM

Blood vessel formation, called *angiogenesis*, starts at the beginning of the third week in the extraembryonic mesoderm of the yolk sac, connecting stalk, and chorion. Blood vessels begin to develop in the embryo about 2 days later (Fig. 3–4A).

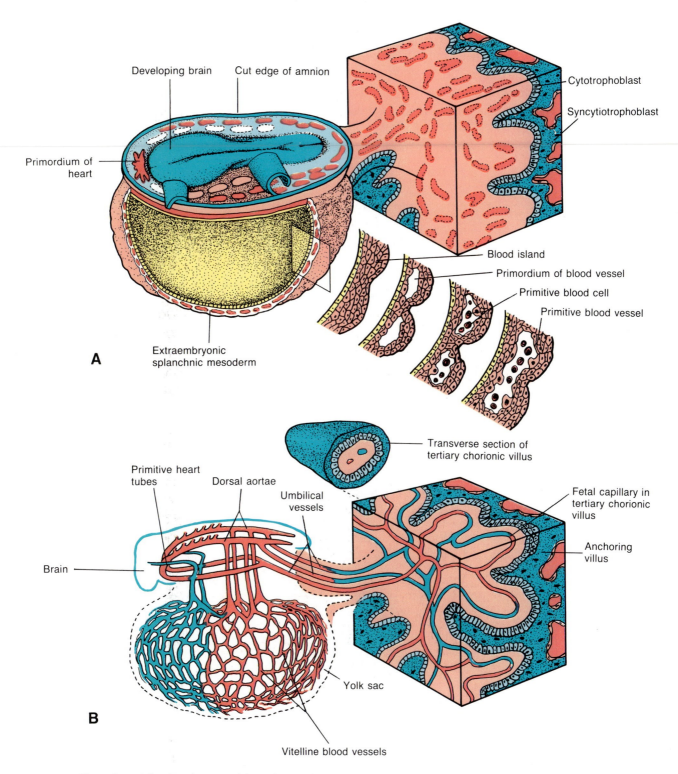

Figure 3–4 Schematic drawings of the embryo and its extraembryonic membranes toward the end of the third week, illustrating formation of blood cells and blood vessels. *A*, the amniotic sac has been cut away to expose the embryo. The clear spaces are the primordia of the intraembryonic coelom, whereas the red spaces are the primordia of the embryonic blood vessels. Part of the yolk sac has also been removed to show how blood islands form in the mesoderm of its walls and give rise to primitive blood cells and blood vessels. *B*, schematic representation of the primitive cardiovascular system in an embryo at the end of the third week, showing its relationship to the placenta and the yolk sac.

The early formation of the cardiovascular system is correlated with the absence of a significant amount of yolk in the ovum and yolk sac. At the end of the second week, embryonic nutrition is obtained from the maternal blood by diffusion through the trophoblast (see Fig. 2–2B). The substances then pass via the extraembryonic coelom and yolk sac to the embryo. As the embryo begins to develop rapidly in the third week, there is an urgent need for vessels to bring nourishment and oxygen to the embryo from the maternal circulation.

Blood vessel formation may be summarized as follows (see Fig. 3–4A):

1. Mesenchymal cells, known as *angioblasts*, aggregate to form isolated masses and cords known as *blood islands*;
2. Cavities appear in these islands;
3. Mesenchymal cells arrange themselves around these cavities to form the *endothelium of primitive blood vessels*;
4. The primitive endothelial vessels fuse to form networks; and
5. Vessels extend into adjacent areas and fuse with other vessels.

Primitive plasma and **blood cells** develop during the third week from the endothelial cells of the vessels in the walls of the yolk sac and allantois. *Blood formation does not begin in the embryo until the fifth week.*

The **primitive heart** is a tubular structure which forms like a large blood vessel from mesenchymal cells in the *cardiogenic area* (see page 128). Paired endocardial *heart tubes* develop before the end of the third week and begin to fuse to form a primitive heart. By the end of the third week, the heart tubes have joined blood vessels in the embryo, connective stalk, chorion, and yolk sac to form a *primitive cardiovascular system* (see Fig. 3–4B). The circulation of blood starts by the end of the third week as the tubular heart begins to beat.

The cardiovascular system is the first organ system to reach a functional state.

DEVELOPMENT OF CHORIONIC VILLI

The primary chorionic villi that started to develop at the end of the second week soon begin to branch. Early in the third week mesenchyme grows into the primary chorionic villi, forming a core of loose connective tissue. The villi at this stage are called *secondary chorionic villi*. Soon some of the mesenchymal cells in the core of the villi begin to differentiate into blood capillaries (see Fig. 3–4A) which soon join to form arteriocapillary-venous networks. As soon as blood vessels have developed in the villi, they are called *tertiary chorionic villi* (see Fig. 3–4B).

The vessels in the chorionic villi soon become connected with the embryonic heart via blood vessels that differentiate in the mesenchyme of the chorion and connecting stalk. By the end of the third week, embryonic blood begins to circulate through the capillaries of the chorionic villi.

Oxygen and nutrients in the maternal blood in the intervillous spaces diffuse through the walls of the villi and enter the fetal capillaries.

Carbon dioxide and waste products diffuse from the blood in the fetal capillaries through the walls of the villi into the maternal blood in the intervillous spaces.

As the tertiary chorionic villi develop, some of their cytotrophoblastic cells proliferate and extend through the syncytiotrophoblastic layer where they join to form a *cytotrophoblastic shell* around the chorionic sac (see Fig. 3–4A and page 46).

This shell attaches the chorionic sac to the endometrium (lining of the uterus). Villi that are attached to the maternal tissues via the cytotrophoblastic shell are called stem villi or *anchoring villi*. By the end of the third week a *primitive placenta* has formed that involves the entire surface of the chorionic sac and the endometrium associated with it.

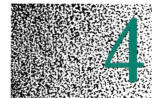

FOURTH TO EIGHTH WEEK OF HUMAN DEVELOPMENT

FOURTH TO EIGHTH WEEK OF HUMAN DEVELOPMENT

The fourth to eighth week constitute a very important period of embryonic development because *the beginnings of all major external and internal structures appear during these five weeks*. By the end of the eighth week, all the main organ systems have begun to develop, but the function of most organs is minimal.

During the fourth week, *folding of the embryo in the median and horizontal planes* converts the flat, trilaminar embryonic disc into a C-shaped, cylindrical embryo (Fig. 4–1). Formation of the head, tail, and lateral folds is a continuous sequence of events that results in a constriction between the embryo and its yolk sac.

During folding, *the dorsal part of the yolk sac is incorporated into the embryo* as the **primitive gut** (see Fig. 4–1E to G).

As the head region of the embryo "swings" or folds ventrally, part of the yolk sac is incorporated into the developing head as the **foregut** (see Fig. 4–1E to G). Owing to folding of the head region, *the oropharyngeal membrane and the heart are carried ventrally*. As a result, the developing brain becomes the most cranial part of the embryo.

As the tail region of the embryo "swings" or folds ventrally, part of the yolk sac is incorporated into the developing caudal region as the **hindgut**. The terminal part of the hindgut soon dilates to form the **cloaca** (see Fig. 4–1G). Owing to folding of the tail region, *the cloacal membrane, allantois, and connecting stalk are carried ventrally* (see Fig. 4–1E to G).

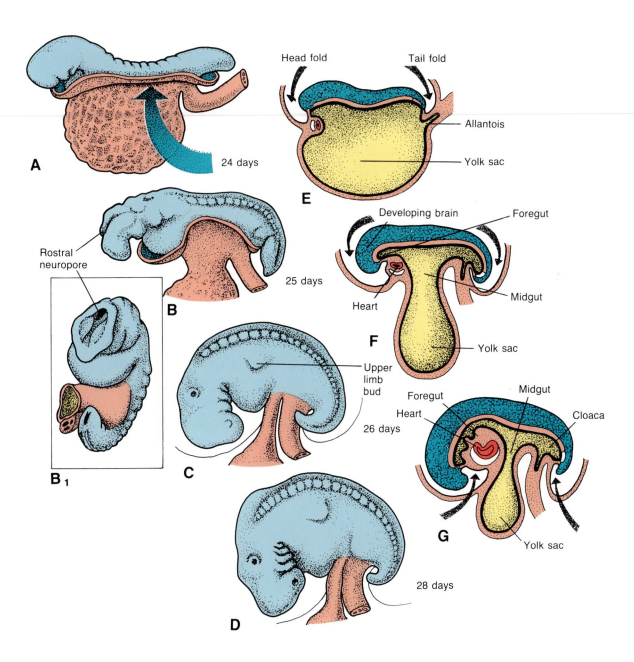

Figure 4–1 Drawings of embryos during the fourth week of development, illustrating folding of the head and tail regions. B_1, demonstrates the open rostral neuropore that is present at 25 days. In the longitudinal sections (E to G), note that the dorsal part of the yolk sac is incorporated into the embryo to form the primitive gut (foregut, midgut, and hindgut).

The folding of the embryo in the horizontal plane incorporates part of the yolk sac into the embryo as the **midgut** (see Figs. 4–1G, and 4–2F). The yolk sac remains attached to the midgut by a narrow *yolk stalk* (see Fig. 4–2G). Folding in the horizontal plane also forms the lateral and ventral body walls (see Fig. 4–2D).

During the fourth to eighth week, the **three germ layers**, derived from the inner cell mass during the third week, *differentiate into various tissues and organs.* The external appearance of the embryo is greatly affected by the formation of the brain, heart, liver, somites, limbs, ears, nose, and eyes. As these structures develop, the appearance of the embryo changes and these characteristics soon mark the embryo as unquestionably human (see Fig. 4–3).

Because the basic organs and systems are formed during the fourth to eighth week, this period constitutes *the most critical period of embryonic development.* Developmental disturbances during this period may give rise to major congenital malformations of the embryo.

HIGHLIGHTS OF THE FOURTH TO EIGHTH WEEK

The following descriptions summarize the main developmental events and changes in external form that occur during this 5-week period.

The Fourth Week

At *the beginning of the fourth week*, the embryo is almost straight and the **somites** produce conspicuous surface elevations (see Fig. 4–2E). At this time the **neural tube** is formed near the middle of the embryo, but it is widely open at the rostral and caudal **neuropores**. The first and second pairs of **branchial arches** are visible and the *otic placodes* (primordia of the internal ears) are recognizable (see Fig. 4–2F and G).

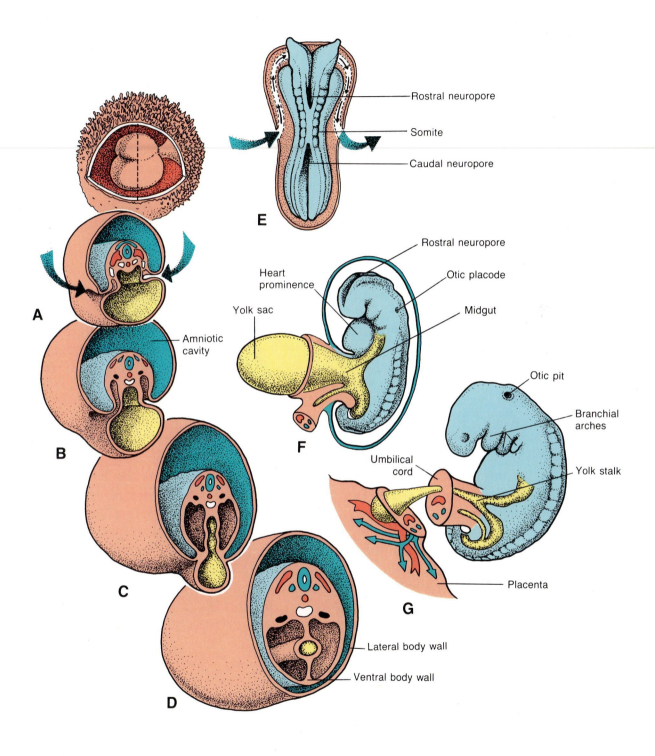

Figure 4–2 Drawings of embryos during the fourth week of development. *A* to *D*, three-dimensional transverse sections of embryos at the plane shown in the drawing at the top left. Note that the dorsal part of the yolk sac in this region is incorporated into the embryo as the midgut. *E*, an embryo (about 22 days) showing the neuropores and the communication between the extraembryonic and intraembryonic coeloms (*arrows*). *F*, the rostral neuropore in this embryo is still open (25 days) and the yolk sac is being incorporated into the embryo. *G*, the rostral neuropore in this embryo is closed (27 days) and the yolk sac is much smaller.

By *the middle of the fourth week*, the embryo is cylindrical and curved owing to folding in the median and horizontal planes (see Figs. 4–1C and 4–2F). The rostral neuropore closes at this time and the **upper limb buds** appear as *small swellings* on the lateral body wall (see Fig. 4–1C). Three pairs of branchial arches are also visible (see Fig. 4–2G) and the heart forms a distinct prominence on the ventral surface of the embryo. Invagination of the otic placodes has formed **otic pits**.

By *the end of the fourth week*, the caudal neuropore has also closed and the embryo has a C-shaped appearance (see Figs. 4–1D and 4–2G). *The upper limb buds have a flipper-like appearance* and the **lower limb buds** appear as *small swellings* on the lateral body wall (Fig. 4–3). Four pairs of branchial arches and *lens placodes* (primordia of the lenses of the eyes) have developed. An *attenuated tail* is a prominent feature of embryos at the end of the fourth week (see Fig. 4–3).

The Fifth Week

Growth of the head is obvious during this week owing to the rapid development of the brain. During the early part of the fifth week, *the upper limbs become paddle-shaped* (see Fig. 4–3). The **cervical sinuses** are now visible. These depressions result from growth of the second branchial arch over the third and fourth pairs of branchial arches.

The Sixth Week

The limbs show considerable regional development during this week, especially the upper limbs (see Fig. 4–3). The elbow and wrist regions are identifiable and the paddle-shaped hand plates have developed ridges, called **digital rays** (finger rays), that indicate the *future digits* (fingers and thumb).

By *the end of the sixth week*, the **foot plates** have appeared and the ankle regions are recognizable. The primordia of the *external acoustic meatus* (auditory or ear canals) and the **external ears** are present. These structures are indicated by small swellings called *auricular hillocks* that develop around the first branchial groove between the first and second branchial arches (see Fig. 4–3).

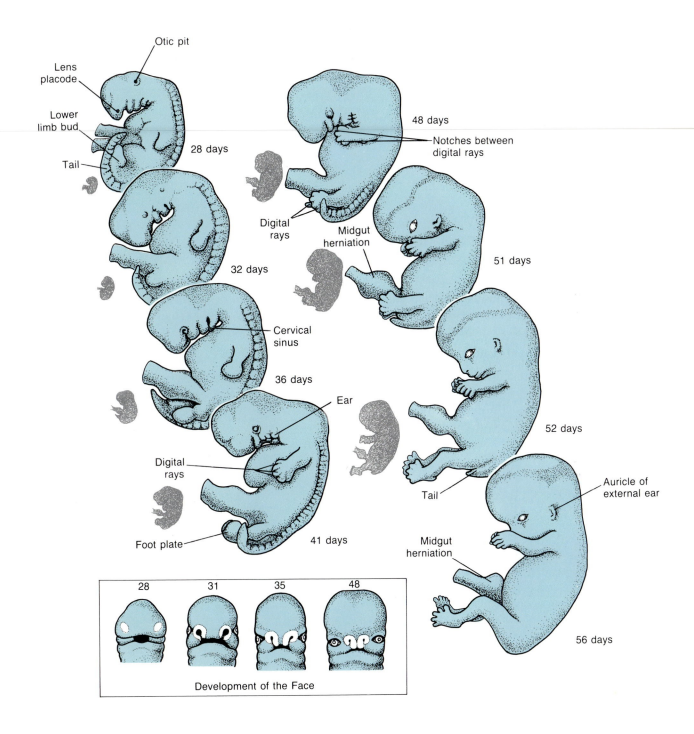

Otic pit

Lens placode

Lower limb bud

Tail

28 days

32 days

Digital rays

Cervical sinus

36 days

Digital rays

Foot plate

41 days

48 days

Notches between digital rays

Midgut herniation

51 days

52 days

Tail

Midgut herniation

Ear

Auricle of external ear

56 days

| 28 | 31 | 35 | 48 |

Development of the Face

Figure 4–3 Drawings of embryos during the embryonic period. The small embryos (*gray*) indicate their actual size. The development of the face is also illustrated (*lower left*). By the end of the eighth week (56 days), the embryo has unquestionably human characteristics. The digits (fingers and toes) are separate and the tail has disappeared.

The Seventh Week

Notches develop between the digital rays in the hand plates that clearly define the future digits (see Fig. 4–3). *Digital rays* (toe rays) appear in the developing feet. The **midgut herniation** is prominent. The disproportionate size of the head is now obvious.

By *the end of the seventh week,* the upper limbs are bent at the elbows and the fingers and thumb are distinct, but they are webbed. By this time, *notches have appeared between the digitial rays in the developing feet.*

The Eighth Week

At *the beginning of the eighth week,* the digits of the hand are short and noticeably webbed (see Fig. 4–3). Distinct notches are visible between the digital rays in the feet. A *stubby tail is still present during the early part of the eighth week,* but it disappears a few days later. By the end of the eighth week, the regions of the limbs are apparent and *the fingers and toes are distinct and separated.*

At the end of the eighth week the embryo has unquestionably human characteristics (see Fig. 4–3). The abdomen still protrudes because the intestines are in the proximal part of the umbilical cord. The eyes are open during most of the eighth week. Towards the end of the week, the eyelids approach each other and may fuse. The auricles of the external ears are beginning to assume their final appearance, but they are still low set on the head. Although the external genitalia have begun to differentiate, *sex differences are not obvious.*

5

NINTH TO THIRTY-EIGHTH WEEK OF HUMAN DEVELOPMENT

NINTH TO THIRTY–EIGHTH WEEK OF HUMAN DEVELOPMENT

The period from the beginning of the ninth week to the end of intrauterine life is known as **the fetal period**. The transition from an embryo to a fetus is neither abrupt nor spectacular, but the name change is made to signify that *the embryo has acquired unmistakable human characteristics.*

Development during the fetal period is primarily concerned with growth of the body and growth and differentiation of the tissues and organs that formed during the embryonic period. The striking change that occurs during the fetal period is the relative slowdown in the growth of the head compared with the rest of the body (Figs. 5–1 and 5–2).

HIGHLIGHTS OF THE FETAL PERIOD

Although there is no formal system of staging for the fetal period, it is helpful to consider the changes that occur in periods of four to five weeks.

Nine to Twelve Weeks

At the beginning of the ninth week, *the head constitutes almost half the crown-rump length of the fetus* (see Fig. 5–1). Subsequently, growth in body length accelerates rapidly, so that by the end of 12 weeks its crown-rump length has more than doubled.

Primary ossification centers appear in the skeleton by the end of this period, especially in the skull and long bones (see Fig. 5–1).

At nine weeks the face is broad, the eyes are widely separated, the ears are low-set on the large head, and the eyelids are fused (see Fig. 5–1). In addition, the legs are short and the thighs are relatively long. By the end of the twelfth week, the upper limbs have almost reached their final relative lengths, but the lower limbs are still not well developed and they are slightly shorter than their final relative lengths. *The fetus begins to move* during the ninth to twelfth week period, but these movements are not felt by the mother.

The external genitalia of males and females are somewhat similar during the ninth week, but their mature fetal form is reached by the end of the twelfth week. Intestinal loops are still visible in the proximal end of the umbilical cord at nine weeks, but they have reentered the abdomen by the beginning of the eleventh week.

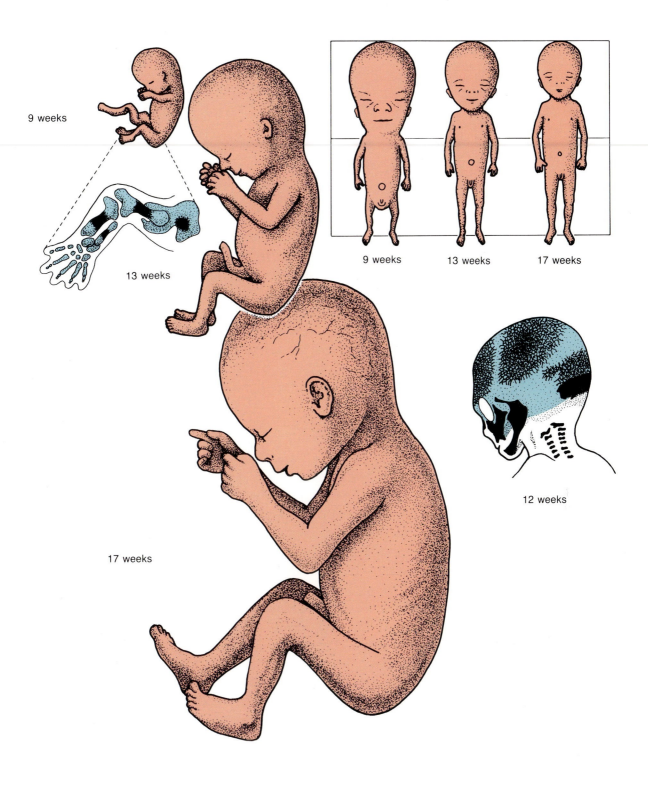

9 weeks

13 weeks

9 weeks   13 weeks   17 weeks

12 weeks

17 weeks

Figure 5–1 Drawings of fetuses at nine, thirteen, and seventeen weeks after fertilization. The spreading areas of intramembranous ossification (*black*) are shown in the flat bones of the skull at 12 weeks. Membranous areas are shown in blue. The developing bones of the face and occipital region are shown in black. Although the primordium of the mandible is originally cartilaginous, the bone shown here has developed by intramembranous ossification of the mesenchyme surrounding Meckel's cartilage in the first branchial arch (see Chapter 9). At the *top right* are drawings illustrating the changing proportions of the body during the fetal period.

At nine weeks, the liver is the major site of **erythropoiesis** (red blood cell production). But by the end of the twelfth week this activity has decreased in the liver and has begun in the spleen.

Urine formation begins during the ninth to twelfth week period and is excreted into the amniotic fluid. The fetus reabsorbs some of this fluid after swallowing it. The waste products in the swallowed fluid pass into the maternal circulation via the placenta.

Thirteen to Sixteen Weeks

Body growth is very rapid during this period (see Figs. 5–1 and 5–2). By 16 weeks the head is relatively small compared with that of the 12-week fetus, and the lower limbs are well developed and have lengthened.

Ossification of the skeleton is now occurring rapidly and many parts of it show clearly on radiographs of the mother's abdomen by the end of this period.

By 16 *weeks the ovaries have differentiated* and many primordial follicles containing oogonia (primitive oocytes or ova) are visible. By the end of this period, the appearance of the fetus is even more human because *its eyes now face anteriorly* rather than anterolaterally. In addition, the auricles of the external ears are close to their definitive positions on the sides of the head.

Seventeen to Twenty Weeks

Although growth of the fetus slows down during this period, growth of the limbs continues until they reach their final relative proportions (see Figs. 5–1 and 5–2). Strong fetal movements, known as **quickening**, are commonly felt by the mother at the beginning of this period. The law usually requires the reporting of the birth of a fetus whose gestational age is 20 weeks (18 weeks after fertilization), or older.

By the end of this period the skin is covered with a cream cheese-like material known as **vernix caseosa**. It consists of a mixture of fatty secretions from the fetal sebaceous glands and dead epidermal cells. The vernix caseosa protects the fetus' skin from abrasions, chapping, and hardening that could result from its exposure to the contaminated amniotic fluid.

The bodies of 20-week fetuses are usually completely covered with fine downy hair called *lanugo*. This hair may help to hold the vernix caseosa on the skin.

Eyebrows and head hair are also visible at 20 weeks (see Fig. 5–2). *Brown fat* forms during the seventeenth to twentieth weeks. This special fat is the site of heat production, particularly in the newborn infant.

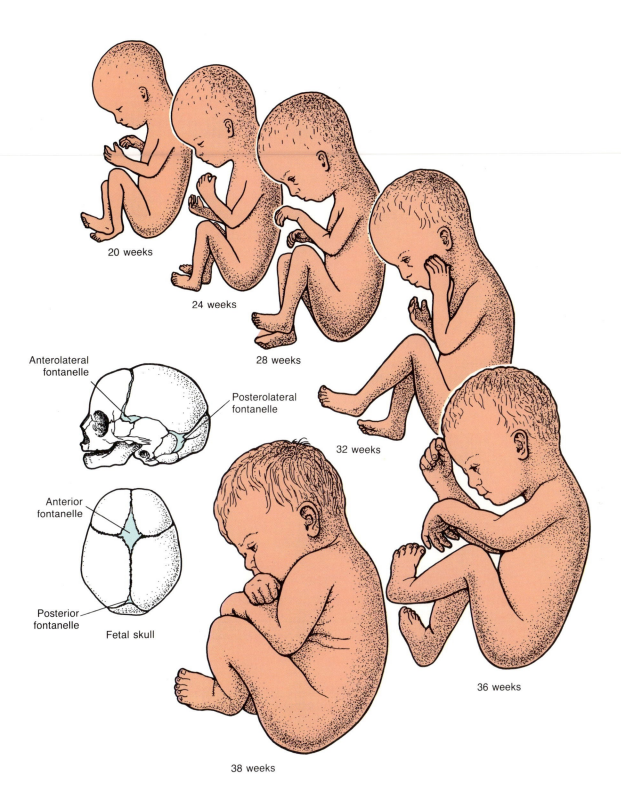

20 weeks

24 weeks

28 weeks

Anterolateral
fontanelle

Posterolateral
fontanelle

Anterior
fontanelle

Posterior
fontanelle

Fetal skull

32 weeks

36 weeks

38 weeks

Figure 5–2 Drawings of fetuses at the ages indicated. Note that some hair is present at 20 weeks and that the eyes are open at 28 weeks. Fetuses born after 32 weeks have a good chance of survival. Note that the flat bones of the fetal skull are separated from each other by sutures (*blue*). In areas where more than two bones meet, the wide sutures are known as fontanelles.

Twenty-One To Twenty-Five Weeks

A substantial weight gain occurs during this period (see Figs. 5–1 and 5–2). Although still somewhat lean, the body of the fetus is now better proportioned. The skin is usually wrinkled and pink to red in fresh specimens because the blood in the capillaries is visible through the very thin skin. The fingernails are well developed at the end of this period, and the toenails have started to develop.

By 24 weeks, the secretory epithelial cells or type II pneumocytes in the interalveolar walls of the lungs have begun to secrete **surfactant**. This substance facilitates expansion of the developing alveoli of the lungs. Consequently, a 22- to 25-week fetus born prematurely may survive if given intensive care, but it usually dies because its lungs are still relatively immature.

Twenty-Six to Twenty-Nine Weeks

Many fetuses born prematurely during this period survive if given intensive care, because their lungs are capable of breathing air. The primitive alveoli and pulmonary vasculature have developed sufficiently to provide adequate gas exchange. In addition, the central nervous system has matured sufficiently to direct rhythmic breathing movements and to control body temperature.

The eyes reopen at the beginning of this period (see Fig. 5–2). Considerable fat forms under the skin so the fetus is not as wrinkled. Erythropoiesis ends in the spleen by 28 weeks and begins in the bone marrow. Toenails are well developed by the end of this period.

Thirty to Thirty-Four Weeks

Normally the *pupillary light reflex* of the eyes can be elicited at 30 weeks. Usually, by the end of this period, the skin is pink and smooth and the upper and lower limbs have a chubby appearance.

Fetuses 32 weeks and older usually survive if born prematurely (see Fig. 5–2).

Thirty-Five to Thirty-Eight Weeks

Fetuses at 35 weeks have a firm grasp and exhibit a spontaneous orientation to light. Most fetuses during this "**finishing period**" are plump (see Fig. 5–2). By 36 weeks, *the circumference of the head and the abdomen are approximately equal.* At the end of this period, the circumference of the abdomen may be greater than that of the head.

Birth usually occurs 266 days or 38 weeks after fertilization. Obstetricians usually report the date of birth as 280 days or 40 weeks after the last menstrual period.

FACTORS INFLUENCING GROWTH OF THE FETUS

Considerable variation exists in the length and weight of fetuses. Most factors influencing fetal growth are genetically determined, but environmental factors may also play an important role. The following maternal factors are known to cause **intrauterine growth retardation:**

1. severe malnutrition;
2. alcohol and drug abuse;
3. heavy cigarette smoking; and
4. placental insufficiency resulting in impaired blood flow and oxygen supply to the fetus.

PRENATAL ASSESSMENT OF THE FETUS

Special techniques are available for assessing the developmental status of a fetus as follows:

1. **Amniocentesis** is the withdrawal of amniotic fluid from the amniotic cavity. It may be analyzed for alpha-fetoprotein, a substance that is highly concentrated in the amniotic fluid when the fetus has a severe **neural tube defect**, such as *spina bifida cystica* or meroanencephaly (absence of most of the brain). The nuclei of cells obtained from amniotic fluid can also be analyzed for **chromosomal abnormalities** (e.g., trisomy 21 that causes the Down syndrome).
2. **Chorionic villi sampling** is also used to obtain fetal tissue for chromosome analysis. This technique can be performed during the seventh and eighth weeks after fertilization, several weeks before amniocentesis is possible.
3. **Ultrasonography** is used to produce images of the fetus and its placenta that can be used to monitor the growth and development of a fetus, especially in high risk pregnancies. Major congenital malformations, such as *hydrocephalus* and *meroanencephaly*, can also be detected by ultrasonography.

Most techniques for determining the prenatal status of a fetus are used in **high risk pregnancies** involving one or more of the following: late maternal age, a history of neural tube defects in the family, and the birth of a previous child with a severe chromosomal abnormality (e.g., trisomy 13 that results in malformation and death of the fetus).

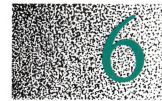

6

PLACENTA AND FETAL MEMBRANES

PLACENTA AND FETAL MEMBRANES

The **primitive placenta** forms during the second week (see page 10). As the walls of the maternal arterioles and venules are eroded by the rapidly proliferating syncytiotrophoblast of the blastocyst, maternal blood seeps in and out of the **lacunar networks** in the syncytiotrophoblast (see Fig. 2–2). Beginning at the end of the second week, cords of cytotrophoblast cells migrate into the finger-like processes of the syncytiotrophoblast, forming **primary chorionic villi** (see Fig. 2–2C).

During the third week, the extraembryonic mesoderm of the **chorion** invades the cytotrophoblastic cores of the primary villi (see page 24), forming **secondary chorionic villi**. By the end of the third week, some mesenchymal cells in the core of each villus differentiate into blood capillaries, forming **tertiary chorionic villi** (see Figs. 6–1A$_1$ and 6–2D). These vessels soon join to form an arterio-capillary-venous network (see Fig. 3–4B). The arteries and veins in the chorionic villi soon connect with blood vessels in the chorion, connecting stalk (future umbilical cord), and embryo (see Fig. 6–1A$_1$).

The endometrium (lining of the uterus) in a pregnant woman is known as the **decidua** which means "cast off." It was so named because it is "cast off" or sloughed off with the placenta after birth. Three regions of the decidua are recognized (see Fig. 6–1B): (1) *decidua basalis*, the region between the blastocyst and the myometrium; (2) *decidua capsularis*, the endometrium that covers the implanted blastocyst and separates it from the uterine cavity; and (3) *decidua parietalis*, all the remaining endometrium (see Fig. 6–1A).

As the embryo and its membranes enlarge, the decidua capsularis is stretched. As a result the chorionic villi on the associated part of the chorionic sac gradually atrophy and disappear (see Fig. 6–1A to C). This villus-free part of the chorionic sac is known as the **smooth chorion** (chorion laeve). Meanwhile, the chorionic villi related to the decidua basalis have increased rapidly in size and complexity (see Fig. 6–1C). This region of the chorionic sac is known as the bushy or **villous chorion** (chorionic frondosum).

STRUCTURE OF THE PLACENTA

The placenta is a fetomaternal organ, because it is formed by both fetal and maternal tissues. By the beginning of the twelfth week, two distinct components of the placenta are recognizable: (1) a **fetal portion** formed by the bushy or *villous chorion*, and (2) a **maternal portion** formed by the *decidua basalis* (see Fig. 6–2C).

The two portions of the placenta are held together by *stem villi* that are often called **anchoring villi** (see Fig. 6–2C) because they are anchored to the decidua

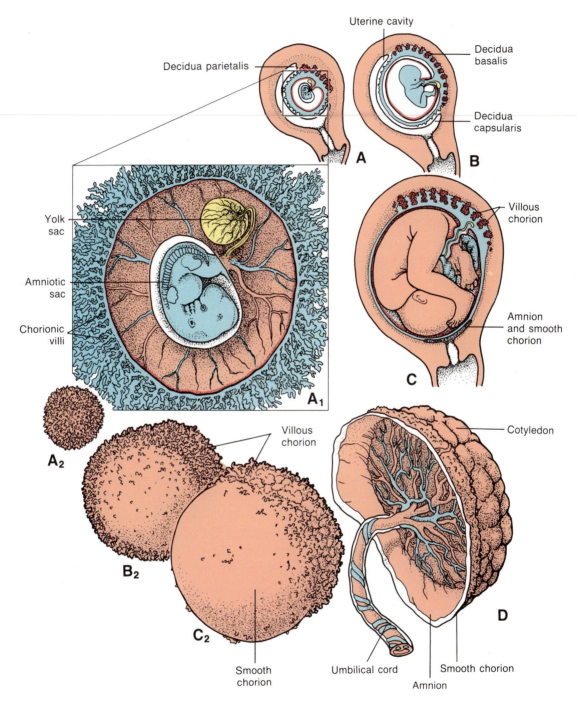

Figure 6–1 Drawings illustrating the relationship of the conceptus (embryo and fetus and their membranes) to the decidua, which is the name given to the pregnant endometrium or lining of the uterus. *A* to *C*, drawings of schematic sagittal sections of the uterus from the fourth to the twenty-second week, which show the changing relations of the fetal membranes to the decidua. A_2, up to the eighth week chorionic villi cover the entire surface of the chorionic sac. B_2, after the eighth week chorionic villi degenerate on that part of the chorionic sac related to the decidua capsularis. This part, devoid of chorionic villi and smooth in appearance, is known as the smooth chorion (C_2). The part of the chorion that retains chorionic villi is known as the villous chorion, and it forms the fetal part of the placenta. *D*, a full-term placenta. Note that the amnion covers the fetal surface of the placenta and forms the epithelial covering of the umbilical cord. Owing to the presence of cotyledons (clumps of main stem chorionic villi), the maternal surface of the placenta has a cobblestone appearance.

basalis by way of the **cytotrophoblastic shell** (see Fig. 6–2D). During erosion of the decidua basalis by the syncytiotrophoblast, large areas of decidual tissue are excavated to form irregular **intervillous spaces** (see Fig. 6–2C). During this erosion of the decidua basalis, parts of the decidua remain as solid projections called **placental septa**. These septa project into the intervillous spaces and divide the placenta into a number of compartments. Each compartment contains a **cotyledon** (see Figs. 6–1D and 6–2B), which consists of several stem villi and their many branches (see Fig. 6–2C).

The Placental Membrane (Placental Barrier). This thin fetal membrane separates the fetal blood in the capillaries of the chorionic villi from the maternal blood in the intervillous spaces (see Fig. 6–2B to D). During the early months of pregnancy, the placental membrane consists of four layers: (1) the fetal capillary epithelium, (2) connective tissue, (3) cytotrophoblast, and (4) syncytiotrophoblast. During the later stages of pregnancy the cytotrophoblast disappears, the syncytiotrophoblast becomes very thin, and the connective tissue becomes greatly reduced. As a result, the placental membrane separating the fetal and maternal blood streams becomes extremely thin (about 1 micron).

THE PLACENTAL CIRCULATION

Maternal Placental Circulation. Oxygenated maternal blood enters the intervillous spaces from the eroded ends of **spiral arteries** in the decidua basalis (see Fig. 6–2B and C). The blood pressure is sufficient to direct the blood towards the **chorionic plate** and to deflect it over the branches of the chorionic villi. The deoxygenated maternal blood leaves the intervillous spaces through openings in the cytotrophoblastic shell and enters numerous thin-walled **endometrial veins** (see Fig. 6–2C). The periodic uterine contractions compress the intervillous spaces, forcing the blood into these branches of the uterine veins.

Fetal Placental Circulation. Deoxygenated fetal blood leaves the fetus in two **umbilical arteries** that pass through the umbilical cord (see Fig. 6–2B). When they reach the fetal surface of the placenta, these vessels divide into many branches which enter the chorionic villi (see Fig. 6–2C). Oxygenated blood returns to the fetus via the venules and veins in the chorionic villi. These join to form the **umbilical vein** in the umbilical cord (see Fig. 6–2C).

FUNCTIONS OF THE PLACENTA

There are six main functions of the placenta.

1. **Respiration**. *Oxygen* in the maternal blood diffuses across the placental membrane into the fetal blood by simple diffusion. *Carbon dioxide* also passes readily in the opposite direction. The placenta, therefore, acts as "the lungs of the fetus."
2. **Nutrition**. Water, inorganic salts, carbohydrates, fats, proteins, and vitamins all pass from the maternal blood through the placental membrane into the fetal blood.

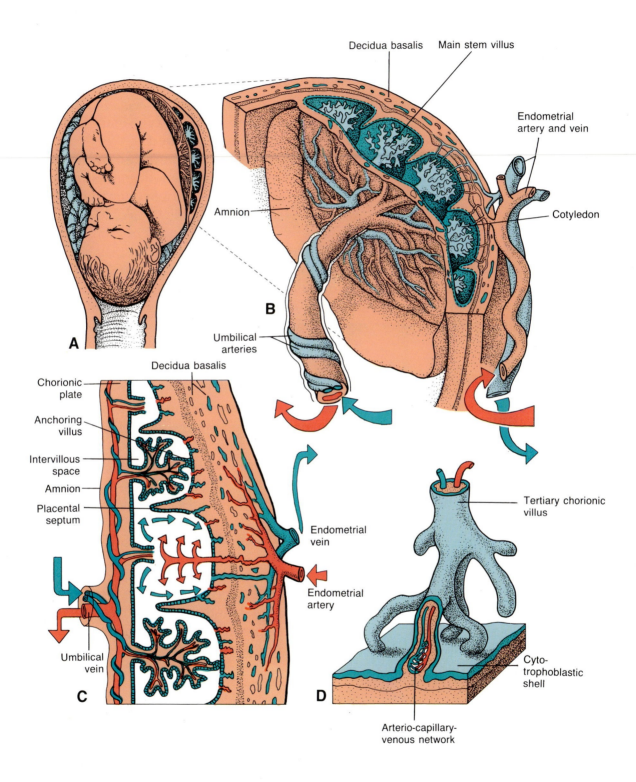

Figure 6–2 Schematic drawings of the fetus and placenta. which illustrate how the placenta supplies oxygen and nutrition to the embryo and removes its waste products. Deoxygenated blood leaves the fetus in the umbilical arteries and enters the placenta where it is oxygenated. Oxygenated blood leaves the placenta in the umbilical vein which enters the fetus via the umbilical cord.

3. **Excretion**. Waste products cross the placental membrane from the fetal blood and enter the maternal blood. They are excreted by the mother's kidneys.

4. **Protection**. Most microorganisms do not cross the placental membrane (e.g., bacteria), but some do (e.g., *Toxoplasma gondii, an intracellular parasite*). There is no appreciable mixture of maternal and fetal blood.

5. **Storage**. Carbohydrates, proteins, calcium, and iron are stored in the placenta and are released into the fetal circulation as required.

6. **Hormonal production**. The following hormones are produced by the syncytiotrophoblast of the placenta: human chorionic gonadotropin, estrogens, progesterone, and human chorionic somatomammotropin (human placental lactogen).

Although the *placental membrane* is often referred to as the *placental barrier*, it does not protect the fetus from many damaging agents such as drugs, poisons, carbon monoxide, and certain viruses (e.g., rubella virus). Once in the fetus, these substances produce congenital malformations (e.g., the rubella virus causes **congenital cataracts**). Such agents are referred to as *teratogens* (see page 59).

MULTIPLE PREGNANCY

The placenta and fetal membranes in multiple pregnancy vary, depending on (1) the derivation of the embryos and their membranes, and (2) when separation of the blastomeres occurs.

The common type of twins is **dizygotic twins (fraternal twins)**. As the adjective "dizygotic" indicates, these infants are *derived from two zygotes* (Fig. 6–3A). Consequently they are associated with two amnions, two chorions, and two placentas that may or may not be fused.

Monozygotic twins (identical twins) are less common, representing about a third of all twins. As the adjective "monozygotic" indicates, they are *derived from one zygote* (see Fig. 6–3B). This type of twins commonly has two amnions, one chorion, and one placenta. Some monozygotic twins have one amnion, one chorion, and one placenta. This results from separation of the embryonic disc into two parts after the amniotic cavity has formed at the beginning of the second week. Other types of multiple birth (triplets, quadruplets, etc.) may be derived from one or more zygotes.

THE YOLK SAC AND ALLANTOIS

The yolk sac and allantois are *vestigial structures* in human embryos. They are however, essential for normal embryonic development because they provide early sites of blood formation. In addition, the dorsal part of the yolk sac is incorporated into the embryo as the **primitive gut** during the fourth week.

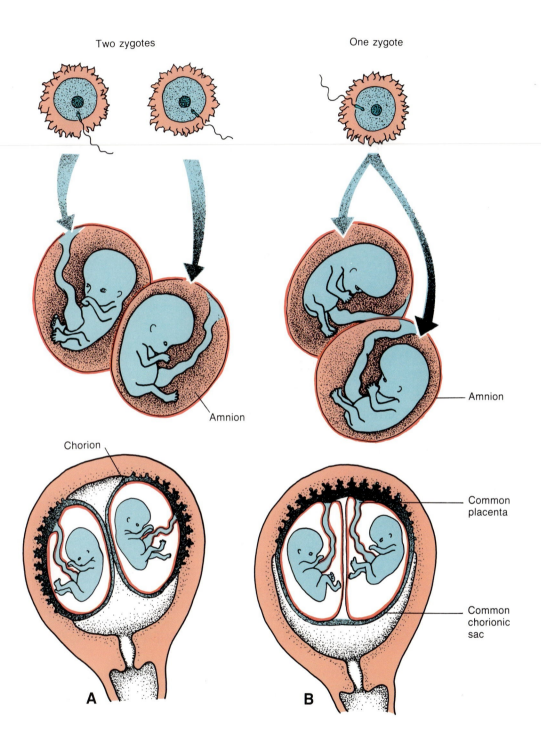

Figure 6–3 Drawings illustrating how twins develop. Twins may originate from two zygotes (A), in which case they are dizygotic or fraternal, or twins may develop from one zygote (B) and be monozygotic or identical. Dizygotic twins may be of the same sex or different sexes. They always have two amnions and two chorions, but the placentas may be fused. Monozygotic twins are of the same sex, usually have separate amnions, and are within the same chorionic sac.

Primordial germ cells also form in the wall of the yolk sac and migrate into the embryo, where they enter the gonads (sex glands) and differentiate into the germ cells (sex cells).

THE AMNIOTIC SAC AND AMNIOTIC FLUID

The amnion forms a sac that encloses the embryo and is attached to it (see Fig. 6–3B). It contains amniotic fluid. It also forms the epithelial covering of the umbilical cord. Most of the amniotic fluid is initially derived from the maternal blood by diffusion across the amnion from the decidua parietalis and the intervillous spaces of the placenta. Later, the fetus makes daily contributions to the amniotic fluid by excreting urine into the amniotic cavity.

Circulation of the Amniotic Fluid.   The water content of amniotic fluid is changed every three hours. Large amounts of amniotic fluid pass through the amnion into the maternal blood, particularly where the amnion is adherent to the fetal surface of the placenta (see Fig. 6–2B).

Amniotic fluid is also swallowed by the fetus and absorbed by the fetal digestive tract. The fluid passes into the fetal blood stream and the waste products in it cross the placental membrane into the maternal blood. Excess water in the fetal blood is excreted by the fetal kidneys and is returned to the amniotic sac.

The amniotic fluid has three main functions. It serves as a protective buffer for the embryo/fetus; provides room for fetal movements; and assists in the regulation of fetal body temperature.

PARTURITION

Parturition or labor is the *birth process* during which the fetus, fetal membranes, and placenta are expelled from the maternal genital tract. Normally parturition occurs about 38 weeks after fertilization. There are three stages of labor: *the first stage (dilatation stage)* ends with complete dilitation of the cervix; *the second stage (expulsion stage)* ends with the delivery of the baby; and *the third stage (placental stage)* ends when the placenta and fetal membranes are expelled after birth.

THE FULL-TERM PLACENTA

The placenta expelled from the uterus after the birth of a baby commonly has a discoid shape, a diameter of 15 to 20 cm, a thickness of 2 to 3 cm, and a weight of 500 to 600 g. The margins of the placenta are continuous with the ruptured amniotic and chorionic sacs (see Fig. 6–1D).

The Maternal Surface of the Placenta.   The characteristic cobblestone appearance of this surface is caused by the **cotyledons** (see Fig. 6–1D) which are composed of several main stem villi and their branches (see Fig. 6–2B). The maternal surface is covered with a thin layer of decidua basalis. However, most of the maternal portion of the placenta remains in the uterus and is expelled with subsequent bleeding.

The Fetal Surface of the Placenta.   The umbilical cord attaches to this surface, often near its center (see Figs. 6–1D and 6–2B and C). The amnion covers the fetal surface and is continuous with the amnion forming the epithelial covering of the umbilical cord. The blood vessels which radiate from the umbilical cord into the chorionic villi and from the villi into the cord, are visible through the transparent amnion.

The Umbilical Cord.   The umbilical cord usually contains two arteries and one vein (see Figs. 6–1D and 6–2B). They are surrounded by mucoid connective tissue (**Wharton's jelly**). The umbilical cord is usually 1 to 2 cm in diameter and 30 to 90 cm in length (average 55 cm). Excessively long or short umbilical cords may be associated with congenital malformations.

HUMAN CONGENITAL MALFORMATIONS

HUMAN CONGENITAL MALFORMATIONS

Congenital malformations (birth defects) are anatomical or structural defects that are present at birth (L. *congenitus*, born with). *Morphogenesis*, the differentiation of cells and tissues that forms the embryo's organs and parts, is an elaborate process and, therefore, it is not surprising that malformations resulting from *dysmorphogenesis* occur (Gr. *dys*, abnormal).

About three percent of all live-born infants have an obvious major malformation. By the end of the first year this figure is doubled to about six percent, owing to the detection of another three percent of infants with malformations that were not obvious at birth. Congenital malformations may be single or multiple and they may be of minor or major clinical significance.

Single minor malformations are present in about 14 percent of newborns. These malformations (e.g., a simian crease in the palm, Fig. 7–1C, and cutaneous ear tags) are of no functional significance, but they alert the clinician to the possible presence of an associated major malformation.

Ninety percent of infants with multiple minor malformations have one or more associated major malformation. Of the three percent of infants that are born with a major congenital malformation, 0.7 percent of them have multiple major malformations (see Fig. 7–1 and Tables 7–1, 7–3, and 7–4).

Major malformations are more common in early embryos (10 to 15 percent) than they are in newborn infants (3 to 6 percent), but most severely abnormal embryos are spontaneously aborted during the first six to eight weeks.

TABLE 7–1 Trisomy of the Autosomes

Chromosomal Aberration	Incidence	Usual Characteristics
Trisomy 21 syndrome (see Fig. 7–1)	1:700	Mental deficiency, brachycephaly (short head), flat nasal bridge; upward slant to palpebral fissures; protruding tongue; simian crease, clinodactyly of 5th finger; congenital heart defects
Trisomy 18 syndrome	1:3,000	Mental deficiency; growth retardation; prominent occiput (back part of head); short sternum; ventricular septal defect of heart; micrognathia (small jaw); low-set malformed ears; flexed fingers, hypoblastic nails; rocker-bottom feet
Trisomy 13 syndrome	1:5,000	Severe central nervous system malformations; mental deficiency; sloping forehead; malformed ears, scalp defects; microphthalmia (small eyes); bilateral cleft lip and/or palate; polydactyly (extra digits); posterior prominence of the heels

TABLE 7–2   **Frequency of the Down Syndrome in Newborn Infants**

Maternal Age*	Frequency
20–24	1/1550
25–29	1/1050
30–34	1/700
35	1/350
37	1/225
39	1/150
41	1/85
43	1/50
45+	1/25

* Based on data from Hook EB. Rates of chromosome abnormalities at different maternal ages. Obstet Gynecol 1981; 58:282.

CAUSES OF HUMAN CONGENITAL MALFORMATIONS

Knowing about the causes of congenital malformations is clinically important because about 20 percent of deaths in the perinatal period are attributed to major developmental abnormalities. The etiology or study of abnormal development and its causes is referred to as **teratology**.

The causes of human congenital malformations are illustrated in Figure 7–2: (1) **genetic factors** (chromosomal aberrations and single gene defects); (2) **environmental factors** (drugs, chemicals, infections, and maternal disease); and (3) **multifactorial inheritance** (interaction of multiple genes at different loci with one or more environmental factors). In Figure 7–2, *note that the causes of 54 percent of congenital malformations are unknown.*

Genetic Causes of Congenital Malformations

It is estimated that genetic factors are involved in over a third of all major congenital malformations (see Fig. 7–2), and cause nearly 85 percent of those with known causes.

Numerical Chromosomal Abnormalities

When chromosomal aberrations are present in the zygote, malformations nearly always develop in the embryo. They are usually severe and often result in the death and spontaneous abortion of the embryo early in the pregnancy.

Numerical aberrations or abnormalities of chromosomes cause about 6 percent of the malformations observed in live-born infants (see Fig. 7–2). Usually these defects arise as the result of *an error in cell division* called **nondisjunction**. During this process two members of a chromosome pair fail to disjoin during the anaphase of cell division, so that both chromosomes pass to the same daughter cell. Nondisjunction may occur during mitosis or at the first or second meiotic divisions during **gametogenesis** (*oogenesis or spermatogenesis*).

Persons with numerical chromosomal abnormalities usually have characteristic *phenotypes* (observable physical characteristics), as demonstrated in the following syndromes (see Fig. 7–1 and Tables 7–1 and 7–3).

Trisomy of the Autosomes.   Trisomy of the autosomes results in different syndromes which are now described (see Table 7–1).

Trisomy 21 Syndrome.   Persons with this chromosomal aberration have *an extra chromosome* 21 (see Fig. 7–1D). The overall incidence of trisomy 21, resulting in the **Down syndrome**, is *one per 700 newborn infants*, but its frequency varies with the age of the mother (see Table 7–2).

The incidence of trisomy 21 at fertilization is greater than at birth, but about 60 percent of the resulting embryos are spontaneously aborted and at least 20 percent of the fetuses are stillborn. The usual physical characteristics or stigmata of persons with the Down syndrome are shown in Figure 7–1 and described in Table 7–1.

Severe mental retardation is the most serious result of trisomy 21. The I.Q. is usually less than 50 and *heart malformations* are present in about 40 percent of cases. A few persons with trisomy 21 are **mosaics** (about 1 percent), usually 46/47, that is, they have a mixture of normal cells with 46 chromosomes and abnormal cells with 47 chromosomes. These individuals have mild stigmata of the Down syndrome and are less retarded than typical persons with trisomy 21.

Trisomy 18 Syndrome.   Individuals with this concurrence of symptoms (see Table 7–1) have *an extra chromosome* 18 (see Fig. 7–1D). This numerical chromosomal abnormality causes the spontaneous abortion of most embryos. Its incidence is about *one per 3,000 newborn infants*. Of those born alive, the mean survival is only two months. As with the Down syndrome, the usual basis of trisomy 18 is nondisjunction.

Trisomy 13 Syndrome.   This severe chromosomal aberration, involving *an extra chromosome* 13 (see Fig. 7–1D), is associated with several major congenital malformations (see Table 7–1). Its incidence is about *one per 5,000 newborn infants*. The condition is lethal in about half the cases during the first month. Death of the others is usual within six months. Most cases of trisomy 13 result from *nondisjunction*, but the cause of about 20 percent of these chromosomal aberrations is *translocation* (the transfer of a segment of one chromosome to another).

Trisomy of the Sex Chromosomes.   The incidence of the common sex chromosomal abnormalities is one per 1,000 (see Table 7–3). As with other trisomies, most of the aberrations result from nondisjunction.

The Klinefelter Syndrome (47, XXY).   Persons with this chromosome complement, *an extra X chromosome*, are characterized by *small testes* owing to hyalinization of the seminiferous tubules (see Table 7–3). These males are infertile. The abnormal testes fail to produce adult levels of testosterone which results in *poorly developed secondary sexual characteristics* and *gynecomastia* or excessive development of male mammary glands (in about 40 percent of cases).

Many of these men are tall and eunuchoid (defective masculinity). As with the Down syndrome, *maternal age is advanced* in these cases. About 15 percent

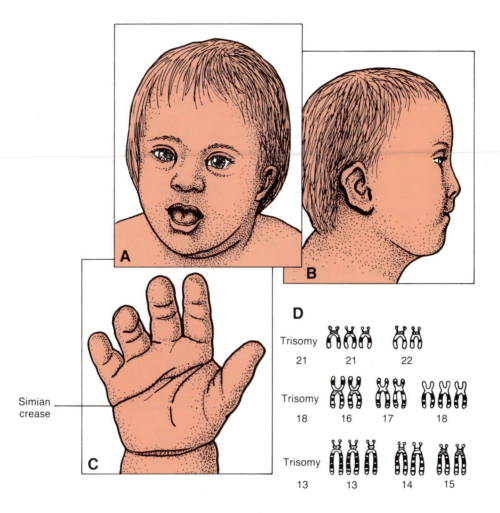

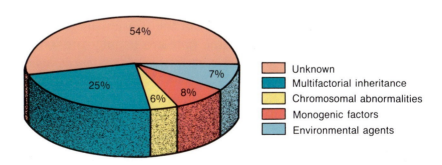

Figure 7–1   *A* and *B*, drawings of a young girl illustrating the typical facial appearance of persons with the Down syndrome (trisomy 21). Observe the flat broad face, oblique palpebral fissures (eye slits), and the large tongue. *C*, drawing of the typical short broad hand, with clinodactyly (lateral deviation of the fourth digit). Note the simian crease that is present in many cases. About one percent of normal persons also have a simian crease. *D*, drawing of some chromosomes in the karyotypes (display of chromosomes) of patients with trisomy 21 (3 chromosomes 21), trisomy 18 (3 chromosomes 18), and trisomy 13 (3 chromosomes 13).

Figure 7–2   A graph illustrating the causes of major congenital malformations. Note that the causes of most of them are unknown and that many malformations are caused by genetic factors (numerical and structural chromosomal abnormalities and mutant genes).

TABLE 7–3   Trisomy of the Sex Chromosomes

Chromosome Complement*	Sex	Incidence	Usual Characteristics
47, XXX	Female	1:1,000	Normal in appearance; usually fertile; 15–25 percent are mildly mentally retarded
47, XXY	Male	1:1,000	Klinefelter syndrome: small testes, hyalinization of seminiferous tubules; aspermatogenesis; often tall with disproportionately long lower limbs. Intelligence is less than in normal siblings.
47, XYY	Male	1:1,000	Normal in appearance; often tall; often exhibit aggressive behavior

*The numbers below designate the total number of chromosomes, including the sex chromosomes shown after the comma.

of males with the Klinefelter syndrome are **mosaics** (46, XY/47, XXY). Mosaics may be fertile.

The XYY Syndrome.   Most males with this chromosomal abnormality, *an extra Y chromosome,* are indistinguishable from normal males (see Table 7–3). Some of these men exhibit aggressive or *criminal behavior* and their intelligence is less than in their normal siblings.

The chromosome abnormality in the XYY syndrome results from nondisjunction during the second meiotic division of spermatogenesis. This produces YY-bearing sperms. There is no apparent paternal age effect.

The XXX Syndrome.   Females with this chromosomal abnormality, *an extra X chromosome,* are normal in appearance, but some of them are mildly mentally retarded (see Table 7–3). They tend to be underweight for their height and to be long-legged.

Most of these women are fertile and their children are usually normal. Nondisjunction at the first meiotic division during oogenesis, or at the second meiotic division during spermatogenesis, is the cause of the XXX chromosomal aberration.

The Turner Syndrome (45, X or Monosomy X).   These females, *missing an X chromosome,* exhibit the following characteristics: *short stature* (125 to 150 cm), *webbing of the neck* (redundant neck skin), *broad chest* with widely spaced nipples, and *cubitus valgus* (reduced carrying angle at the elbow).

The incidence of monosomy X (Turner syndrome) is *one per 2,500 newborn infants,* but its frequency in embryos is much higher; however, about 97 percent of them abort spontaneously. The external genitalia are juvenile and the internal sexual organs are also female, but the ovaries are often only streaks of connective tissue. Axillary and pubic hair are usually present, but sparse.

Monosomy X (Turner syndrome) results from nondisjunction during gametogenesis in either parent. About 40 percent of females with the Turner syndrome are mosaics (e.g., 45,X/46, XX). Their stigmata of the syndrome are less than in the usual cases and their intelligence is normal or slightly reduced.

Structural Chromosomal Abnormalities

Aberrations of chromosome structure result from *chromosome breakage,* followed by reconstitution in an abnormal combination. Chromosome breaks may

TABLE 7-4 Human Teratogens: Environmental Factors Known to Cause Congenital Malformations

Agent	Common Congenital Malformations
DRUGS	
Alcohol	Growth and mental retardation, microcephaly, and facial abnormalities
Aminopterin and methotrexate (Folic acid deficiency)	Hydrocephalus; growth and mental retardation
Androgens and high doses of masculinizing progestogens	Masculinization of the external genitalia of female fetuses
Hydantoin (Dilantin)	Growth retardation, microcephaly, and mental retardation
Lithium carbonate	Cardiac defects
Retinoic acid and high doses of vitamin A	Craniofacial abnormalities and neural tube defects (meroanencephaly and spina bifida)
Tetracycline	Darkly stained teeth; hypoplasia of enamel
Thalidomide	Limb reduction deformities (amelia and meromelia)
Trimethadione	Developmental delay, V-shaped eyebrows, low-set ears and cleft lip and/or palate
Warfarin	Hypoplasia of nasal cartilage; CNS defects
CHEMICALS	
Methylmercury	Cerebral atrophy, spasticity, seizures, and mental retardation
PCBs	Growth retardation; skin discoloration
INFECTIOUS AGENTS	
Cytomegalovirus	Growth and mental retardation; hearing loss
Herpes simplex virus	Microcephaly, microphthalmia, and retinal dysplasia
Rubella virus	Cataracts, deafness, and heart defects
Toxoplasma gondii	Blindness, mental retardation, and microcephaly
Treponema pallidum (syphilis)	Abnormal teeth and bones, microcephaly, and mental retardation
Varicella (chickenpox)	Skin scarring, muscle atrophy, and mental retardation
Venezuelan equine encephalitis	Cataracts; brain destruction
OTHER FACTORS	
Iodine deficiency	Goiter; growth and mental retardation
Ionizing radiation (high levels)	Microcephaly, mental retardation, and skeletal malformation
Maternal phenylketonuria	Microcephaly; mental retardation

*Based on Sever JL. Brent RL. eds. Teratogen update: environmentally induced birth defect risks, New York: Alan R Liss, 1986, and Moore KL. The developing human. Clinically oriented embryology. 4th ed. Philadelphia: WB Saunders, 1988.

be induced by a wide variety of agents, such as *ionizing radiation*, viral infections, drugs, and chemicals. Although many structural chromosomal abnormalities have been detected, the only ones that are likely to be transmitted from parent to child result from **inversion** (a chromosomal aberration in which a segment of a chromosome is reversed end-to-end), and from **translocation** (the transfer of a segment of one chromosome to another chromosome). The transfer usually results in no loss of DNA, hence the individual is usually normal. However the children of these balanced carriers of a chromosomal aberration may be abnormal.

The loss of a portion of a chromosome following a chromosome break is called a **deletion.** The resulting structurally abnormal chromosome lacks the genetic information that is in the lost fragment. The common example of a chromosome deletion in humans is loss of the short arm of chromosome 5. This results in the **cri du chat syndrome**. It was given this name because of the resemblance of the cry of an affected infant to the mewing of a cat. These persons have *microcephaly* (small head), *abnormal facies* (unusual facial appearance), and *severe mental retardation*.

Malformations Caused by Mutant Genes

In monogenic or single-gene disorders, *a single major error in the genetic constitution (genotype) is the basis of the congenital malformations*. New hereditary variations arise by **mutation.** The new gene, or the person who carries it, is called a **mutant**.

A mutation is an error in the replication of DNA that involves a loss or a change in the function of a gene. Most mutations are deleterious; some are lethal. Probably 8.0 percent of congenital malformations are caused by monogenic or single gene defects (see Fig. 7–2).

The rate of gene mutation is increased by a number of environmental agents (e.g., large doses of radiation and chemicals, especially carcinogenic [cancer-inducing] ones).

Examples of *dominantly inherited congenital malformations* are **achondroplasia** (small stature with short limbs and large head) and **polydactyly** (extra digits). Achondroplasia is an autosomal dominant disorder that often results from a new mutation.

Environmental Causes of Congenital Malformations

About seven percent of congenital malformations are caused by environmental agents known as *teratogens* (see Fig. 7–2 and Table 7–4).

Human teratogens are environmental agents that produce or raise the incidence of congenital malformations. The organs and parts of an embryo are most sensitive to teratogenic agents during their periods of rapid differentiation (see Fig. 7–3).

The known human teratogens (see Table 7–4) are *drugs* (e.g., thalidomide), *chemicals* (e.g., methylmercury), *infectious agents* (e.g., rubella virus), and high levels of *ionizing radiation* (e.g., from atomic accidents).

Teratogens present during the first two weeks of development have no teratogenic action or their effects are so severe that they cause the death and spontaneous abortion of the embryo.

The stage of development of the embryo or fetus determines its susceptibility to teratogens (see Fig. 7–3). When the embryo's parts and organs are forming (i.e., during the *organogenetic period*, particularly from *days 15 to 60*), teratogenic agents may cause major congenital malformations (see Fig. 7–3 and Table 7–4). However, the critical period for brain growth and development is from the third to sixteenth weeks and mental development may be severely affected by teratogens, such as *cytomegalovirus* and large doses of *ionizing radiation*, even in the perinatal and infantile periods.

The period of greatest sensitivity for radiation damage to the brain leading to severe mental retardation is from eight to 16 weeks after fertilization.

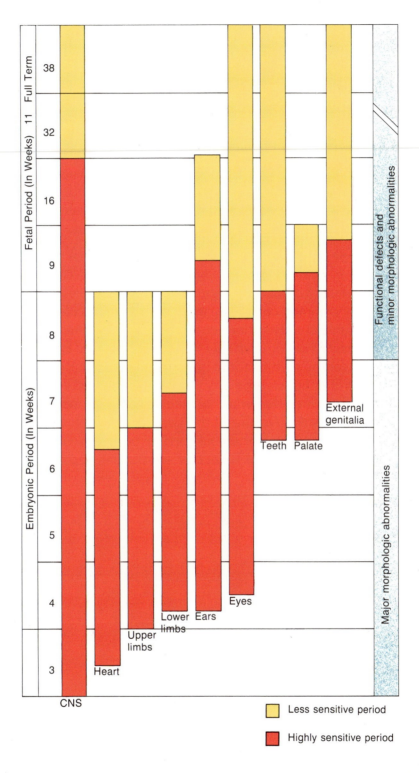

Figure 7–3 Schematic illustration showing the critical periods during human development. Note that each organ or part of the embryo has a critical period (shown in red) during which its development may be deranged. Thereafter, there is a period (shown in yellow) when functional and minor malformations may be produced, e.g., the central nervous system (CNS) is vulnerable to teratogenic agents up to the end of the sixteenth week. (Modified from Moore KL. The developing human. Clinically oriented embryology. 4th ed. Philadelphia: WB Saunders, 1988.)

The best known and one of the most potent teratogens is *thalidomide*. This drug caused *major limb malformations* and various other abnormalities in infants whose mothers took the drug during the critical period of their embryos' development (see Fig. 7–3), especially 24 to 36 days after fertilization. Other known human teratogens are shown in Table 7–4 which lists the common congenital malformations that are produced by these teratogenic agents.

During the **fetal period**, teratogens may produce *minor morphological defects* (e.g., slight enlargement of the clitoris, and mild to *severe functional abnormalities*, particularly of the brain and eye (e.g., mental retardation and blindness). For example, high doses of *ionizing radiation* and major *alcohol abuse* during the fetal period, are likely to cause *mental retardation*. Tetracyclines, androgens, and infectious agents can also produce birth defects during the fetal period, as described in Table 7–4.

Multifactorial Causes of Congenital Malformations

Most congenital malformations with known causes result from multifactorial inheritance (see Fig. 7–2). Many common congenital malformations (**cleft lip** with or without **cleft palate**) have familial distributions consistent with multifactorial inheritance. *These malformations result from the combined effect of the genetic and environmental factors.* Malformations caused by multifactorial inheritance are usually single major abnormalities such as cleft lip, cleft palate, **neural tube defects** (e.g., meroanencephaly, partial absence of the brain, or anencephaly, absence of the brain, and spina bifida, a defective closure of the vertebral arch through which there is a protrusion of the meninges or spinal cord or both), and **congenital heart malformations** (e.g., atrial septal defect or ventricular septal defect).

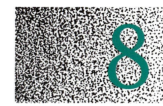

EMBRYONIC BODY CAVITIES, PRIMITIVE MESENTERIES, AND DIAPHRAGM

EMBRYONIC BODY CAVITIES, PRIMITIVE MESENTERIES, AND DIAPHRAGM

The embryonic body cavities, *pericardial, pleural,* and *peritoneal,* are formed by partitioning of the **primitive intraembryonic coelom.** The intraembryonic coelom begins developing in the lateral and cardiogenic mesoderm during the third week (see page 22). By the early fourth week, the intraembryonic coelom on each side communicates across the midline, just cranial to the *oropharyngeal membrane,* forming a horseshoe-shaped cavity (Fig. 8–1A). The portion of the coelom that lies cranially, called the *pericardial coelom,* will form the **pericardial cavity** around the heart. The limbs of the horseshoe-shaped intraembryonic coelom form the *pleural* and *peritoneal cavities* around the lungs and abdominopelvic organs, respectively (Fig. 8–1C).

FOLDING OF THE EMBRYO

As the head folds ventrally early in the fourth week, the future pericardial cavity comes to lie ventral to the developing gut (see Fig. 8–1B). Part of the embryonic mesoderm that was initially cranial to the developing pericardial cavity comes to lie caudal to it and ventral to the developing gut. This mass of mesoderm, called the **septum transversum,** is the primordium of the *central tendon of the diaphragm* (Fig. 8–2E).

Initially the intraembryonic coelom is continuous on each side of the embryo with the extraembryonic coelom (see Fig. 8–1A). This communication is important because the midgut must herniate into the umbilical cord in this region owing to the small size of the abdominal cavity during the embryonic period (see page 34). The midgut develops within the umbilical cord into the small intestine and part of the large intestine. When the intestines return to the abdomen during the tenth week, the connection between the intraembryonic and extraembryonic coeloms is obliterated.

During folding of the embryo in the horizontal plane (see Figs. 4–2 and 8–1C), the limbs of the horseshoe-shaped intraembryonic coelom are brought together on the ventral surface of the embryo. Initially, the embryonic body cavity is continuous, but the location of its future three regions can be recognized: (1) a large *pericardial cavity;* (2) two relatively small *pericardioperitoneal canals* connecting the pericardial and peritoneal cavities; and, (3) a large *peritoneal cavity.*

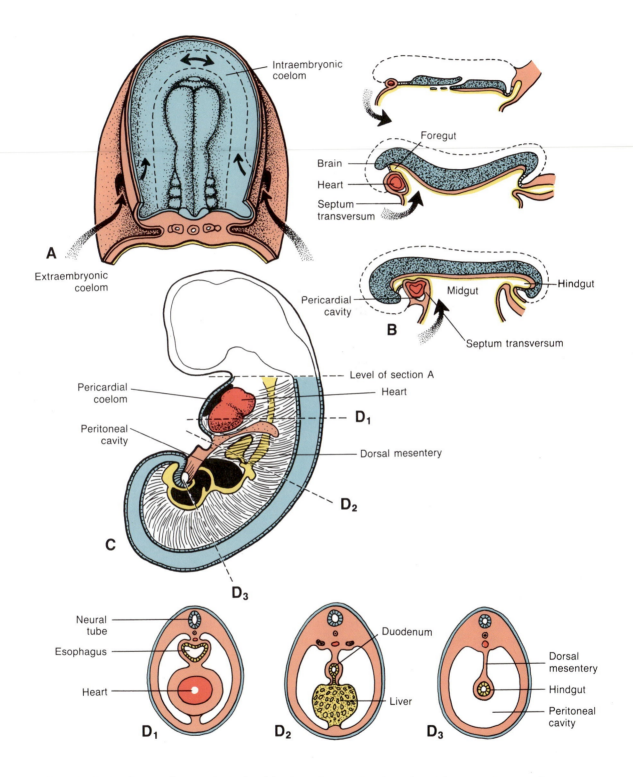

Figure 8–1 *A,* schematic drawing of a 21-day-old embryo showing the relationship of the intraembryonic celom to the extraembryonic celom. The arrows indicate the site of communication of these parts of the celom at this stage. *B,* sketches of sagittal sections of embryos illustrating folding of the head and tail regions of the embryo during the fourth week. Note that as the head folds, the heart and septum transversum are carried ventrally. Also note that during this process, part of the yolk sac is incorporated into the embryo as the primitive gut. *C,* an illustration showing the primitive mesenteries of the embryo as viewed from the left side; *D₁* to *D₃,* diagrammatic transverse sections of the embryo through the levels indicated in *C.*

Initially the dorsal and ventral mesenteries divide the peritoneal cavity into right and left halves (Fig. 8–1D$_1$ and D$_2$), but the ventral mesentery soon disappears (see Fig. 8–1C and D$_3$), except where it is attached to the caudal part of the foregut (the primordium of the stomach and the first part of the duodenum). Following the disappearance of the ventral mesentery, the peritoneal cavity becomes a large continuous space (see Fig. 8–1D$_2$).

DIVISION OF THE INTRAEMBRYONIC COELOM INTO THE BODY CAVITIES

As the **lung buds** (primordia of the lungs) develop, they grow into the pericardioperitoneal canals (see Fig. 8–2B). During this process two pairs of membranous ridges are produced in the lateral walls of each canal (see Fig. 8–2A). The cranial ridges, called **pleuropericardial membranes**, are located superior to the developing lungs. The caudal ridges, called **pleuroperitoneal membranes**, are located inferior to them. As the pleuropericardial membranes enlarge, they gradually separate the pericardial cavity from the pleural cavities.

The Pleuropericardial Membranes (see Fig. 8–2A). These membranes contain the *common cardinal veins* which enter the embryonic heart. Initially, the pleuropericardial membranes project into the cranial ends of the pericardioperitoneal canals. With subsequent growth of the common cardinal veins, descent of the heart, and expansion of the pleural cavities, the pleuropericardial membranes become mesentery-like folds extending from the lateral thoracic wall to the median plane. By the seventh week, the pleuropericardial membranes fuse with the mesoderm ventral to the esophagus. This fusion separates the pericardial cavity from the pleural cavities.

The Pleuroperitoneal Membranes (see Fig. 8–2A to E). As these membranous folds in the caudal ends of the pericardioperitoneal canals enlarge, they gradually separate the pleural cavities from the peritoneal cavity. They enlarge as the developing lungs and pleural cavities invade the body wall. During the sixth week, the pleuroperitoneal membranes extend medially until their free edges fuse with the dorsal mesentery of the esophagus and the septum transversum (see Fig. 8–2B). This separates the pleural cavities from the peritoneal cavity. Closure of the pleuroperitoneal openings is completed as primitive muscle cells from the body wall grow into the pleuroperitoneal membranes (see Fig. 8–2E).

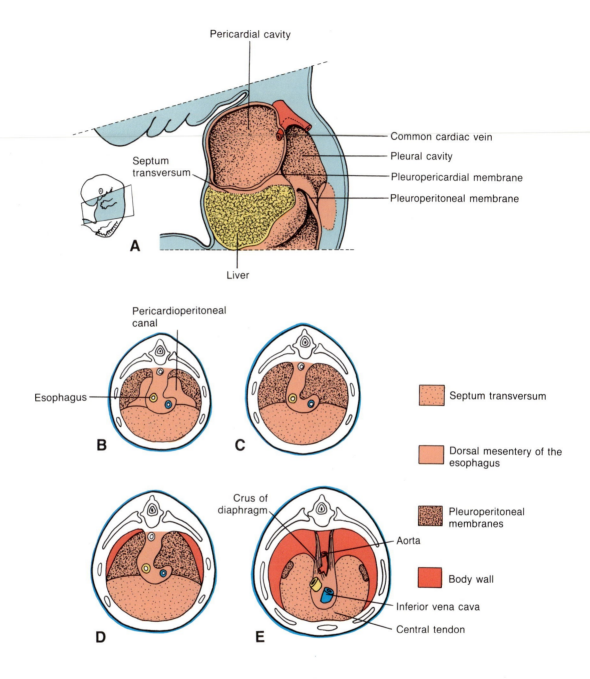

Figure 8-2 *A,* sagittal section of the portion of the embryo indicated in the sketch at the left. The heart and lung have been removed. Observe the pleuropericardial and pleuroperitoneal membranes that are separating the embryonic body cavities. *B* to *E,* diagrammatic transverse sections of embryos at 5 to 8 weeks illustrating the development of the diaphragm. Note that the diaphragm develops from four structures: septum transversum, mesentery of the esophagus, pleuroperitoneal membranes, and body wall.

DEVELOPMENT OF THE THORACOABDOMINAL DIAPHRAGM

As its name implies, this diaphragm separates the thoracic and abdominal cavities. The diaphragm develops from the four structures described below.

1. **The Septum Transversum** (see Figs. 8–1B and 8–2).   This transverse septum of mesoderm forms the *central tendon* of the diaphragm. The septum transversum fuses with the mesenchyme ventral to the esophagus and with the pleuroperitoneal membranes.

2. **The Pleuroperitoneal Membranes** (see Fig. 8–2).   These membranous folds fuse with the dorsal mesentery of the esophagus and the septum transversum, completing the partition between the thoracic and abdominal cavities and forming the primitive diaphragm. Although the pleuroperitoneal membranes form large portions of the primitive diaphragm, they represent relatively small portions of the definitive diaphragm (see Fig. 8–2E).

3. **The Dorsal Mesentery of the Esophagus** (see Fig. 8–2B).   This double layer of peritoneum forms the median portion of the diaphragm. The *crura of the diaphragm* develop from muscle fibers that grow into the dorsal mesentery of the esophagus during the ninth to twelfth weeks (see Fig. 8–2E).

4. **The Body Wall** (see Fig. 8–2D).   The lungs and pleural cavities enlarge and invade the body wall. During this process, the tissue is divided into two layers: an outer layer that becomes the body wall and an inner layer that forms the peripheral part of the diaphragm.

Positional Changes of the Diaphragm

During the fourth week the septum transversum, the first indication of the diaphragm, lies opposite the third, fourth, and fifth **cervical somites**. During the fifth week, myoblasts (developing muscle cells) from these somites migrate into the developing diaphragm, bringing their nerves with them from the cervical region. Consequently, the phrenic nerves that supply the diaphragm come from *cervical roots three, four, and five.* These twigs join on each side to form the **phrenic nerve**. Owing to the embryonic origin of the phrenic nerves, the definitive nerves have a long course through the thorax (about 30 centimeters) to innervate the diaphragm.

Unequal growth of the dorsal part of the embryo's body results in the apparent migration or "descent" of the diaphragm. By the sixth week the developing diaphragm is at the level of the thoracic somites; the phrenic nerves now have a descending course. As the diaphragm "moves" relatively further caudally, these nerves are correspondingly lengthened. By the beginning of the eighth week, the dorsal part of the diaphragm lies at the level of the first lumbar vertebra.

The developmental origin of the diaphragm explains its nerve supply. The phrenic nerves supply the entire motor innervation to the diaphragm and most of the sensory innervation. The peripheral region of the diaphragm, which develops from the body wall (see Fig. 8–2E), receives sensory nerves from the lower six or seven intercostal nerves.

Congenital Diaphragmatic Hernia

Posterolateral defect of the diaphragm (Fig. 8–3A) is the only relatively common congenital malformation of the diaphragm. It occurs once in every 2,000 newborn infants. The large defect in the diaphragm results in the herniation of the abdominal contents into the thoracic cavity (see Fig. 8–3B).

Congenital posterolateral defect of the diaphragm results from the defective formation and/or fusion of the pleuroperitoneal membrane with dorsal mesentery of the esophagus and the septum transversum (see Fig. 8–2B to E). The defect, usually unilateral, commonly consists of a large opening in the posterolateral region of the diaphragm (see Fig. 8–3A).

A posterolateral defect of the diaphragm occurs five times *more often on the left side* than on the right side. This likely results from the earlier closure of the right pleuroperitoneal opening, owing to the presence of the large embryonic liver (see page 102).

Normally, the pleuroperitoneal membranes fuse with the other diaphragmatic components by the beginning of the seventh week (see Fig. 8–2E). If a pleuroperitoneal membrane is unfused when the intestines return to the abdomen from the umbilical cord during the tenth week, the intestines usually pass into the thorax. Often the stomach and spleen also herniate into the thorax. In unusual cases, the liver and kidneys may enter the thoracic cavity displacing the lungs and heart. These thoracic intestines usually dilate at birth with swallowed air, compromising the function of the heart and lungs.

If there are abdominal viscera in the thoracic cavity at birth, *the initiation of respiration is usually impaired.* Because the abdominal organs are most often in the left side of the thorax, the heart and mediastinum are usually displaced to the right. *The lungs are often hypoplastic* and greatly reduced in size. Their retarded growth is caused by a lack of room for them to develop and expand normally. After the hernia is reduced (repositioned), the affected lung is usually aerated and achieves its normal size. After the hernia is reduced, the defect in the diaphragm is repaired.

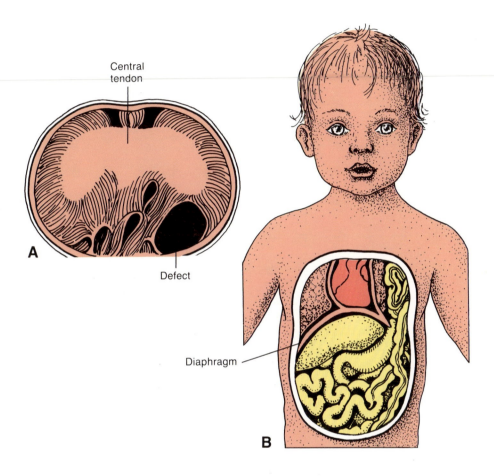

Figure 8–3 *A*, drawing of a diaphragm with a large posterolateral defect resulting from abnormal formation and/or fusion of the pleuroperitoneal membrane on the left side with the mesoesophagus and the septum transversum. *B*, a "window" has been drawn on the thorax and abdomen to show the herniation of the intestine into the thorax through a posterolateral defect in the left side of the diaphragm, similar to that illustrated in *A*. Note that the heart is displaced to the right and that the left lung is compressed.

BRANCHIAL APPARATUS AND HEAD AND NECK

BRANCHIAL APPARATUS AND HEAD AND NECK

During the early part of the embryonic period, the human embryo bears little resemblance to a human being, owing to the presence of the **branchial apparatus** consisting of: (1) **branchial arches** (pharyngeal arches), (2) **pharyngeal pouches**, (3) **branchial grooves** (branchial clefts), and (4) **branchial membranes** (closing membranes). The adjective "*branchial*" is derived from the Greek word, *branchia*, meaning "gill." Although the human embryo never develops gills, it possesses an ancestral branchial apparatus (Fig. 9–1). By the end of the embryonic period, these primitive structures either become rearranged and adapted to new functions or they disappear.

THE BRANCHIAL APPARATUS

Development of The Branchial Arches

The characteristic external feature of the head and neck area of a 4-week-old embryo is the series of branchial arches that are disposed more or less dorsoventrally, and are separated from each other by branchial grooves.

Four branchial arches are visible on the surface (see Fig. 9–1A) and are numbered craniocaudally. The fifth and sixth branchial arches are small and cannot be seen on the surface.

The **first branchial arch**, often referred to as the **mandibular arch**, is large. A *maxillary prominence* (maxillary swelling) grows cranially from its dorsal end, inferior to the developing eye. The maxillary prominence is important in the development of the face (see Figs. 9–1B and 9–4). Another process of the first branchial arch, called the *mandibular prominence*, is also involved in the development of the face, especially in the formation of the lower lip and mandibular region.

Externally the surface ectoderm dips between adjacent branchial arches to form **branchial grooves** (see Fig. 9–1D). Internally the endoderm of the primitive pharynx bulges between the branchial arches to form **pharyngeal pouches** (see Fig. 9–1C). The branchial arches support the lateral walls of the cranial part of the foregut, called the **primitive pharynx**, from which the pharyngeal pouches evaginate. The ectoderm of the branchial grooves and the endoderm of the pharyngeal pouches approach each other between the branchial arches to form **branchial membranes** (see Fig. 9–1D).

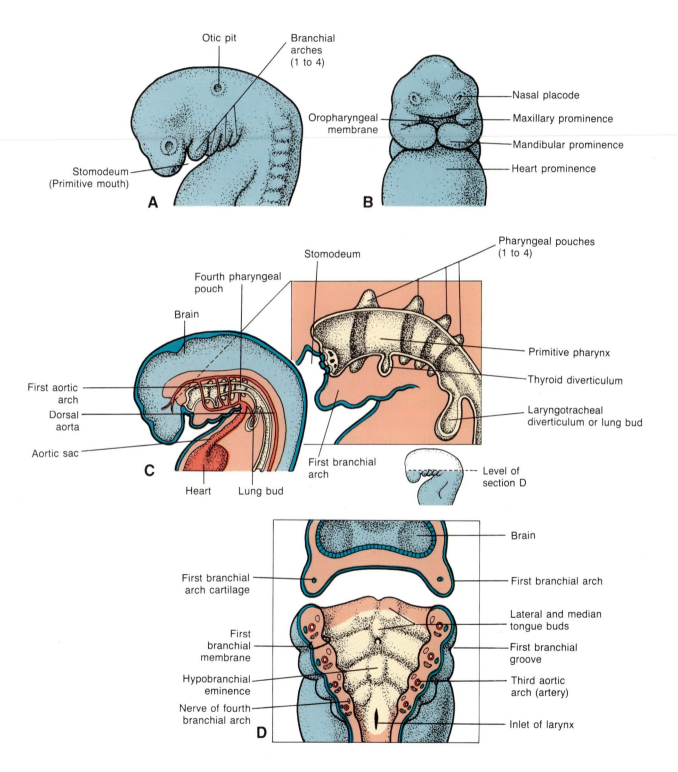

Figure 9–1 Drawings illustrating the branchial apparatus in human embryos during the fourth week. *A*, lateral view at 28 days; *B*, frontal view at 24 days; *C*, schematic lateral view of a sagittal section of a 4-week embryo, illustrating the pharyngeal pouches, aortic arches, and primitive heart; *D*, horizontal section through the cranial end of the embryo shown in C. Note that the branchial apparatus consists of branchial arches, branchial grooves, branchial membranes, and pharyngeal pouches.

The *primitive mouth* initially appears as a slight depression of the surface ectoderm called the **stomodeum** (see Fig. 9–1A). At first the stomodeum is separated from the primitive pharynx by a bilaminar membrane called the **oropharyngeal membrane** (see Fig. 9–1B). It is composed of ectoderm externally and endoderm internally. This membrane ruptures at 24 to 26 days, bringing the primitive gut (primordium of the digestive tract) into communication with the amniotic cavity (see Fig. 9–4A).

Branchial Arch Components

Each branchial arch consists of *mesenchyme* derived from the lateral mesoderm and the **neural crest** (see page 21). This mesenchyme gives rise to muscles, cartilages, bones, and blood vessels. The nerves grow into the arches from the brain.

The Skeletal Components of the Branchial Arches (Fig. 9–2A). Some mesenchymal cells in each branchial arch aggregate to form a longitudinal condensation of cells which is transformed into a *branchial arch cartilage* (see Figs. 9–1D and 9–2A).

The **first branchial arch cartilage** (*Meckel's cartilage*) indicates the position of the future mandible. Two small auditory ossicles (middle ear bones), the *malleus* and *incus*, develop by *endochondral ossification* of the dorsal end of the first branchial arch cartilage. A fibrous remnant of this cartilage forms the **sphenomandibular ligament** (see Fig. 9–2B). The remainder of the first arch cartilage disappears almost completely.

The mandible develops mainly by intramembranous ossification around the first branchial arch cartilages as the latter disappear (see Fig. 9–2B).

The **second branchial arch cartilage** is sometimes called *Reichert's cartilage*. Endochondral ossification of its dorsal end gives rise to the **stapes**, the third ossicle of the middle ear (see Fig. 9–2B). The **styloid process** also develops from the second arch cartilage, as does the *stylohyoid ligament*, the lesser cornu (L. horn), and the *superior part of the body of the* **hyoid bone** (see Fig. 9–2B).

Most of the cartilaginous components of the other branchial arches disappear, but small parts of them remain. The ventral ends of the third pair of branchial arch cartilages form the *inferior part of the body of the hyoid bone and its greater cornua* (horns). The fourth and sixth branchial arches form the cartilages of the larynx, with the exception of the epiglottis (see Fig. 9–2B).

The Muscle Components of the Branchial Arches (see Fig. 9–2C). The mesenchyme in the branchial arches also forms striated muscles. The developing muscle cells (*myoblasts*) migrate to various parts of the head and neck from the branchial arches, where they form the muscles of mastication and facial expression (Fig. 9–2D), but they retain their original nerve supply (Table 9–1).

The Arteries of the Branchial Arches (see Fig. 9–1C). Each branchial arch contains an artery, called an *aortic arch*, that joins the *aortic sac* of the primitive heart ventrally and a *dorsal aorta* dorsally.

The **aortic arches** are not all present at the same time. By the time the sixth pair have developed, the first two pairs of aortic arches have degenerated. The only aortic arches that remain in an altered form in the adult are the third, fourth, and sixth (see Fig. 13–2).

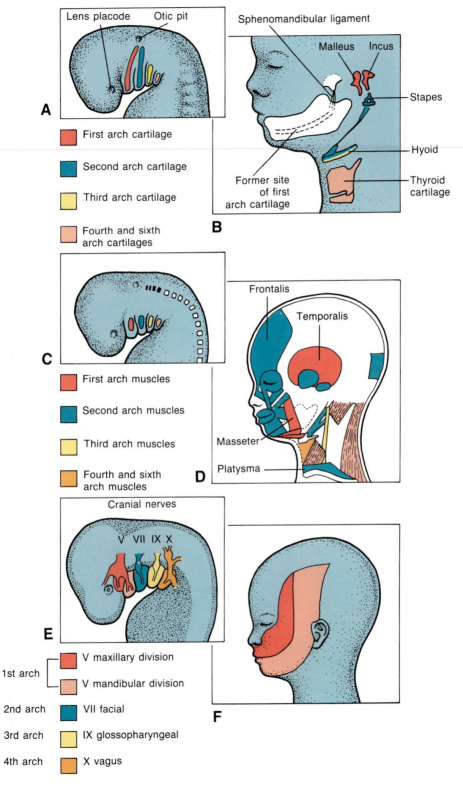

Lens placode   Otic pit

A

First arch cartilage

Second arch cartilage

Third arch cartilage

Fourth and sixth arch cartilages

Sphenomandibular ligament

Malleus   Incus

Stapes

Former site of first arch cartilage

Hyoid

Thyroid cartilage

B

C

First arch muscles

Second arch muscles

Third arch muscles

Fourth and sixth arch muscles

Frontalis

Temporalis

Masseter

Platysma

D

Cranial nerves

V VII IX X

E

1st arch   V maxillary division

V mandibular division

2nd arch   VII facial

3rd arch   IX glossopharyngeal

4th arch   X vagus

F

Figure 9–2   A, schematic drawing of 4-week embryo, illustrating the location of the branchial arch cartilages; B, schematic drawing of a 20-week fetus, illustrating the derivatives or the cartilages derived from the branchial arches; C, drawing of the head of a 4-week-old embryo illustrating the muscle masses in the branchial arches; D, schematic sketch of the head of a 20-week fetus showing the muscles derived from muscle masses in the branchial arches; E, sketch of a 4-week embryo showing the branchial nerves; F, sketch of a lateral view of the head of a 20-week fetus, illustrating the distribution of the two caudal branches of the first branchial nerve (CN V).

The Nerves of the Branchial Arches (see Figs. 9–1D and 9–2E).   The nerves that supply the branchial arches have only a short distance to travel from the brain.

The *fifth cranial nerve* (**trigeminal nerve**, *CN V*) supplies the skin covering the part of the face derived from the first branchial arch, via its maxillary and mandibular divisions (see Fig. 9–2D). The *seventh cranial nerve* (**facial nerve**, CN VII) supplies the muscles derived from the first branchial arch (see Table 9–1). The nerve of the third branchial arch is the *ninth cranial nerve* (**glossopharyngeal nerve**, CN IX). It supplies one muscle (see Fig. 9–2B) and the pharynx. Two branches of the *tenth cranial nerve* (**vagus nerve**, CN X) supply the remaining branchial arches. The superior laryngeal nerve supplies derivatives of the fourth branchial arch and the recurrent laryngeal nerve supplies those in the sixth branchial arch (see Table 9–1).

Other Derivatives of the Branchial Arches (see Figs. 9–2F and 9–3 to 9–5).   The branchial arches, particularly the first and second ones, contribute extensively to the formation of the *face, external ears, neck, mouth, nasal cavities, larynx, palate* and *pharynx*. Six small elevations develop at the dorsal ends of the first and second branchial arches, where they surround the opening of the first branchial groove. These elevations (auricular hillocks) gradually fuse to form the *auricle* (pinna) of the external ear (see Fig. 9–4B) which surrounds the *external acoustic meatus*, a derivative of the first branchial groove (see Fig. 9–3C).

During the fifth week, the second branchial arches enlarge and overgrow the third and fourth branchial arches, forming ectodermal depressions known as **cervical sinuses** (see Fig. 9–4B). These sinuses normally disappear as the external surface of the neck forms.

THE PHARYNGEAL POUCHES

The branchial arches are separated internally by pharyngeal pouches (see Fig. 9–1C) that are located caudal to the arches with corresponding numbers.

Derivatives of the Pharyngeal Pouches (see Fig. 9–3).   The *first pharyngeal pouch* enlarges and develops into a **tubotympanic recess**. This outgrowth becomes the *auditory tube* and the *tympanic cavity* (middle ear cavity).

The cavity of the *second pharyngeal pouch* is largely obliterated as the *palatine tonsil* develops (see Fig. 9–3C), but part of it remains as the **intratonsillar cleft** (tonsillar fossa). The endoderm of the second pharyngeal pouch forms the surface epithelium of the tonsil and the lining of its crypts. The mesenchyme around this pouch differentiates into lymphoid tissue which becomes part of the tonsil.

The endoderm of the dorsal parts of the *third pharyngeal pouches* differentiates into the *inferior parathyroid glands* (see Fig. 9–3B), whereas their ventral parts unite to form the **thymus** (see Fig. 9–3C and D).

The endoderm of the dorsal parts of the *fourth pharyngeal pouches* differentiates into the **superior parathyroid glands**, whereas their ventral parts develop into the *ultimobranchial bodies* (see Fig. 9–3C). These primitive bodies fuse with

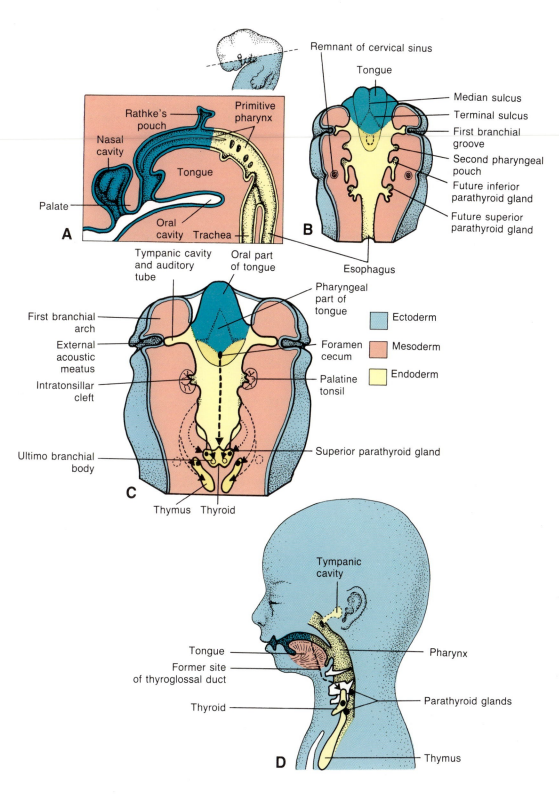

Figure 9–3 Schematic drawings illustrating the derivation of the pharyngeal pouches. *A,* longitudinal section of the head of a 6-week embryo; *B,* horizontal section of the head of the embryo shown in *A,* showing early differentiation of the pharyngeal pouches. *C,* similar horizontal section of a 7-week embryo. *D,* schematic sagittal section of a 20-week fetal head and neck, showing the adult derivation of the pharyngeal pouches and the descent of the thyroid gland from the tongue (*broken line*).

TABLE 9–1   Structures Derived from Branchial Arch Components*

Arch	Nerve	Muscles	Skeletal Structures	Ligaments
First (Mandibular)	Trigeminal† (V)	Muscle of mastication‡ Mylohyoid and anterior belly of digastric Tensor tympani Tensor veli palatini	Malleus Incus	Anterior ligament of malleus Sphenomandibular ligament
Second (Hyoid)	Facial (VII)	Muscles of facial expressions§ Stapedius Stylohyoid Posterior belly of digastric	Stapes Styloid process Lesser cornua of the hyoid Superior part of the hyoid bone	Stylohyoid ligament
Third	Glossopharyngeal (IX)	Stylopharyngeus	Greater cornua of the hyoid Inferior part of body of the hyoid bone	
Fourth and Sixth**	Superior laryngeal branch of vagus (X) Recurrent laryngeal branch of vagus (X)	Cricothyroid Levator veli palatini Constrictors of pharynx Intrinsic muscles of larynx Striated muscles of the esophagus	Thyroid cartilage Cricoid cartilage Arytenoid cartilage Corniculate cartilage Cuneiform cartilage	

* The derivatives of the aortic arches are described in Chapter 13.
† The ophthalmic division does not supply any branchial components.
‡ Temporalis, masseter, medial, and lateral pterygoids.
§ Buccinator, auricularis, frontalis, platysma, orbicularis oris, and orbicularis oculi.
** The fifth branchial arch is often absent. When present, it is rudimentary and usually has no recognizable cartilage. The cartilaginous components of the fourth and sixth arches fuse to form the cartilages of the larynx, as listed.

the thyroid gland (see Fig. 9–3C) and disseminate within it to give rise to the *parafollicular cells* (C cells) of the thyroid gland which produce *calcitonin*, a blood calcium-lowering hormone that is involved in the regulation of the normal calcium level in body fluids.

Branchial Malformations

Most congenital malformations of the head and neck originate during transformation of the branchial apparatus into its adult derivatives. Many of them result from remnants of the branchial apparatus that normally disappear as the adult structures develop. Malformations associated with the branchial apparatus are uncommon, but two of them are clinically important: *first arch malformations* and *remnants of the cervical sinus.*

The First Arch Syndrome. This designation is used for abnormalities that result from *abnormal development of structures derived from the first branchial arch.* This syndrome is believed to result from insufficient migration of cranial neural crest cells into the first branchial arch during the fourth week. The two main manifestations of the first arch syndrome are: **mandibulofacial dysostosis** or *Treacher Collins syndrome* (small mandible, malar hypoplasia, and malformed ears), and the *Pierre Robin syndrome* (small mandible and cleft palate).

Persistence of the Cervical Sinus.   If the cervical sinus (see Fig. 9–4B) does not completely obliterate during formation of the neck, a **branchial cyst** may develop from remnants of it in the neck (see Fig. 9–2B). These cysts are usually *located in the side of the neck along the anterior border of the sternocleidomastoid muscle.* If the persistent cervical sinus is connected with the surface through a narrow duct, it is referred to as an external **branchial sinus**.

Development of the Thyroid Gland

The thyroid gland begins as a downgrowth from the floor of the primitive pharynx (see Fig. 9–1C). This **thyroid diverticulum** soon becomes a bilobed mass of cells that descends in the neck (see Fig. 9–3C). This diverticulum temporarily retains its connection with the tongue by a long **thyroglossal duct**. This duct normally disappears before the end of the embryonic period, but its cranial opening persists as the **foramen cecum** of the adult tongue.

Development of the Tongue

The oral part (anterior two-thirds) of the tongue (see Figs. 9–3C and 10–2C) develops from two *distal tongue buds* (lateral lingual swellings) and a *median tongue bud* (tuberculum impar). These buds result from proliferation of mesenchyme in the first pair of branchial arches (see Fig. 9–1D). The distal tongue buds increase rapidly in size, merge with each other, and overgrow the median tongue bud. The plane of fusion of the distal tongue buds is indicated externally on the tongue by the *median sulcus* and internally by the *median septum* (see Fig. 9–3B).

The pharyngeal part (posterior third) of the tongue (see Figs. 9–3C and 10–2C) develops from two structures: the **copula** and **hypobranchial eminence** (see Fig. 9–1D). These swellings result from proliferation of mesenchyme in the second, third, and fourth pairs of branchial arches. As the tongue develops, the copula is overgrown by the hypobranchial eminence; as a result, the posterior third of the tongue develops from the cranial part of the hypobranchial eminence.

The line of fusion of the oral and pharyngeal parts of the tongue is roughly indicated in the adult by the V-shaped groove, called the *terminal sulcus* (see Fig. 9–3B). The **foramen cecum**, the remnant of the proximal end of the thyroglossal duct, is located at the apex of the terminal sulcus (see Fig. 9–3C).

Development of the Face

The face develops from five primordia (see Fig. 9–4A). The **frontonasal prominence** (swelling) constitutes the cranial boundary of the stomodeum or primitive mouth (see Fig. 9–4B); the paired **maxillary prominences** of the first branchial arch form the lateral boundaries, and the paired **mandibular prominences** of the same arch constitute the caudal boundary.

Thickenings of the surface ectoderm, called **nasal placodes**, develop on each side of the frontonasal prominence (Fig. 9–4A). Horseshoe-shaped ridges develop around these placodes, called the **medial and lateral nasal prominences** (swellings). As a result, the nasal placodes lie in the floor of depressions known as **nasal pits** (see Fig. 9–4C).

Between the fifth and eighth weeks, *the maxillary prominences increase in size and grow medially,* moving the medial nasal prominences toward the median plane. The groove between the lateral nasal prominence and the maxillary prominence disappears as these prominences merge (see Fig. 9–4D).

The upper lip is formed by the merging of the maxillary prominences with the medial nasal prominences. The lateral nasal prominences do not form part of the upper lip; they form the alae (sides) of the nose. When the medial nasal prominences merge, they form an **intermaxillary segment** composed of three parts: (1) a *labial component* which forms the **philtrum** of the upper lip (see Fig. 9–4D); (2) a *maxillary component* that will be associated with the four incisor teeth (see Fig. 9–5F); and (3) a *palatal component* which becomes the primary palate (see Fig. 9–5C).

The **mandibular prominences** grow medially and begin to merge with each other by the end of the fourth week (see Fig. 9–4A). They form the *lower lip, chin,* and *mandible* (see Fig. 9–4B to D).

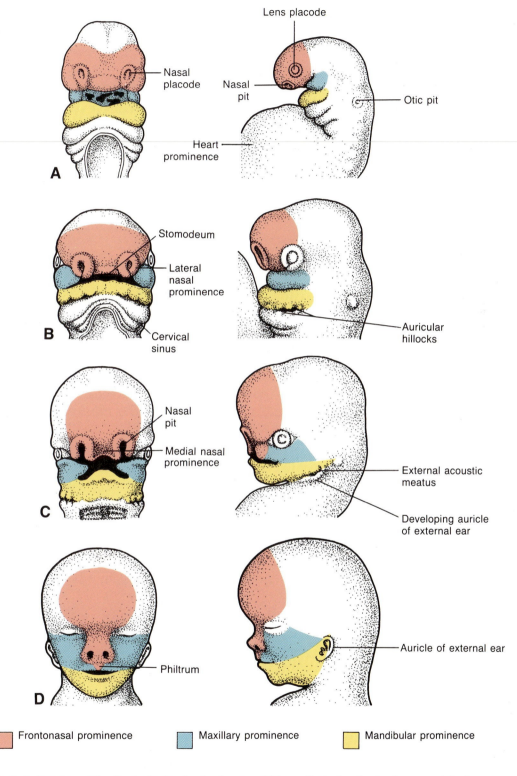

Figure 9-4   Drawings of the developing heads of embryos and fetuses, illustrating the development of the face. *A*, 28 days; *B*, 33 days; *C*, 40 days; *D*, 10 weeks. Left side, frontal views; right side, lateral views.

Development of the Palate

The palate develops from three primordia. The anterior part is derived from the wedge-shaped **primary palate**, known as the **median palatine process** (see Fig. 9–5A). The posterior part of the palate, representing most of the definitive palate, is derived from two shelf-like outgrowths from the internal surfaces of the maxillary prominences, called the **lateral palatine processes** (see Fig. 9–5B).

The **secondary palate** develops as the lateral palatine processes grow medially during the seventh week and fuse with each other in the median plane. The lateral palatine processes also fuse anteriorly with the median palatine process (see Figs. 9–5B to D). As these fusions occur, the nasal septum grows inferiorly and fuses with the palate. The *incisive canal* indicates the division between the parts of the palate derived from the primary and secondary palates (see Fig. 9–5D).

Cleft Lip and Cleft Palate

The most common and important of all congenital malformations of the face are **cleft lip and cleft palate**. These malformations may occur separately or in combination. *Clefts involving the upper lip, with or without cleft palate, occur about once in 1,000 births,* but their frequency varies widely among ethnic groups.

Cleft Lip. *Unilateral cleft lip* is caused by an arrest of mesenchymal proliferation that results in failure of the maxillary prominence on the affected side to merge with the intermaxillary segment formed by the medial nasal prominences.

Bilateral cleft lip is caused by an arrest of mesenchymal proliferation that results in failure of the maxillary prominences on both sides to merge with the intermaxillary segment formed by the medial nasal prominences (see Fig. 9–5E).

Cleft Palate. Minor clefts involve only the uvula (see Fig. 9–5C and D), but most clefts extend through the soft and/or hard regions of the palate. The embryologic basis of posterior clefts of the palate is failure of the lateral palatine processes to fuse with each other, with the nasal septum, and/or with the median palatine process. The clefts may be unilateral or bilateral, and they may or may not be associated with cleft lip.

Causes of Cleft Lip and Cleft Palate. Most cases of cleft lip and cleft palate result from *multifactorial inheritance* (i.e., they are determined by multiple factors, genetic and non-genetic). Teratogenic factors (see page 60) are known to interfere with the number of neural crest cells that migrate into the embryonic facial primordia. If the number of cells is insufficient, a deficiency of mesenchyme results that causes clefting of the lip and/or palate.

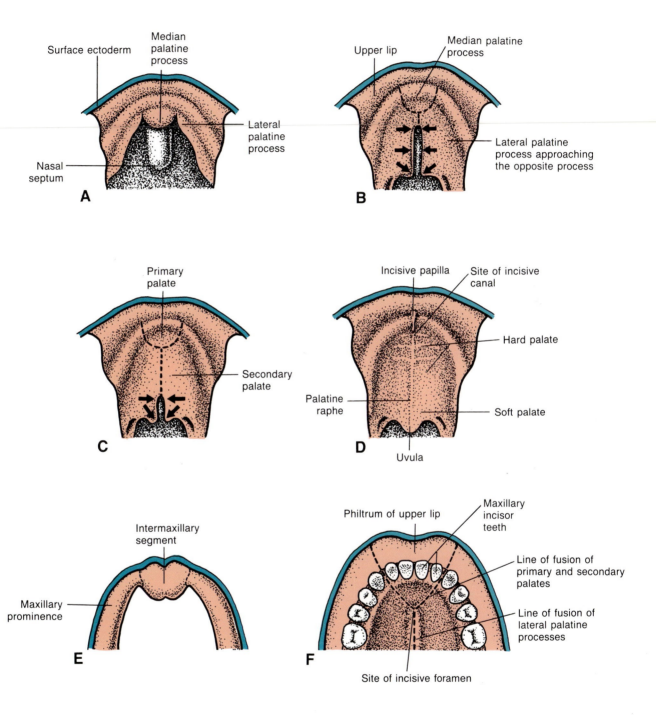

Figure 9–5 Drawing of the roof of the mouth of embryos from the sixth to the twelfth week, illustrating development of the palate. Note that the palate forms from two primorida: the primary palate and the secondary palate. Failure of these parts to fuse results in cleft palate. Note that the intermaxillary segment (shown in *E*) gives rise to (1) the philtrum of the upper lip (also see Fig. 9–4*D*); (2) the premaxillary part of the maxilla that lodges the incisor teeth; and (3) the primary palate (shown in *C*).

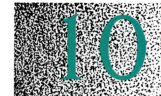

RESPIRATORY SYSTEM

RESPIRATORY SYSTEM

The development of most of the upper respiratory system (the nose, nasopharynx, and oropharynx) is described in Chapter 9. The primordium of the lower respiratory system appears early in the fourth week as a longitudinal groove in the median plane of the floor of the *primitive pharynx*, just caudal to the pharyngeal pouches (Fig. 10–1A and B). This **laryngotracheal groove** produces a ridge on the external surface of the primitive pharynx.

As the embryo develops, the laryngotracheal groove deepens and evaginates to form a **laryngotracheal diverticulum** (see Fig. 10–1E). As this outgrowth extends caudally into the splanchnic mesenchyme, its distal end enlarges to form a globular **lung bud** (see Fig. 10–1F). The endoderm of the laryngotracheal diverticulum (yellow) gives rise to the epithelium of the larynx and trachea, the secretory epithelial cells of the tracheal glands, the epithelium of the bronchi and bronchioles, and the pulmonary lining epithelium. The connective tissue, cartilage, and smooth muscle of these structures develop from the splanchnic mesenchyme (red) surrounding the laryngotracheal diverticulum.

The laryngotracheal diverticulum is separated from the foregut by longitudinal **tracheoesophageal folds** that develop (see Fig. 10–1H) and fuse to form a partition known as the **tracheoesophageal septum** (see Fig. 10–1I). This septum divides the foregut into a ventral portion, called the **laryngotracheal tube** (the primordium of the larynx, trachea, bronchi, and lungs), and a dorsal portion, the **esophagus** (see Fig. 10–1J).

THE LOWER RESPIRATORY SYSTEM
Development of the Larynx

The opening of the laryngotracheal tube into the primitive pharynx (see Fig. 10–1C) becomes the **inlet of the larynx** or laryngeal aditus (Fig. 10–2). The epithelium of the mucous membrane lining the larynx differentiates from the endoderm lining the cranial end of the laryngotracheal tube. The laryngeal cartilages are derived from those in *the fourth and sixth pairs of branchial arches* (see Figs. 9–2B, 10–1C, and Table 9–1).

The mesenchyme around the cranial end of the laryngotracheal tube proliferates rapidly, producing paired **arytenoid swellings** (see Fig. 10–2A). As these swellings grow rostrally toward the tongue, they convert the slit-like laryngeal opening into a T-shaped aperture, called the **inlet of the larynx** (see Fig. 10–2B and C).

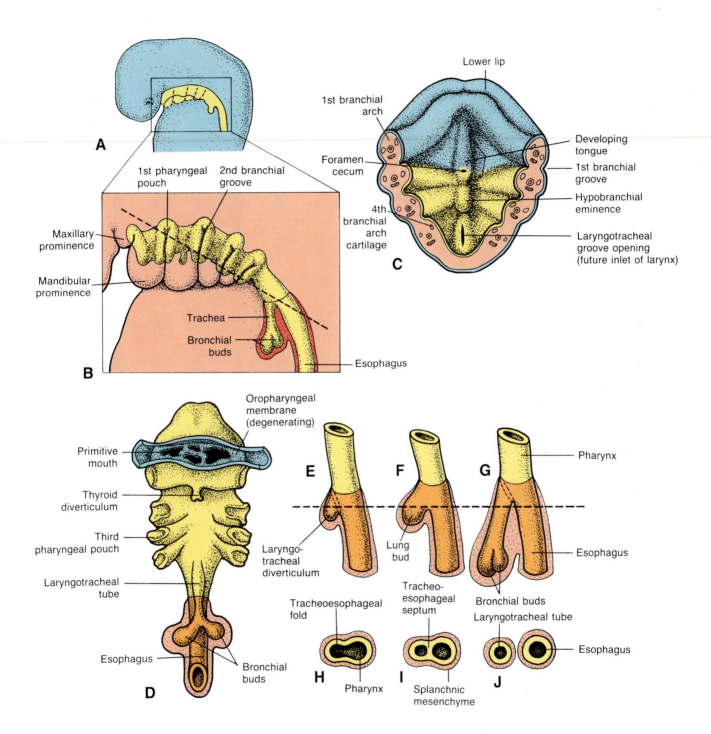

Figure 10–1 Drawings illustrating early development of the lower respiratory system. *A*, diagrammatic sagittal section of the head of a 26-day-old embryo showing the laryngotracheal diverticulum; *B*, enlargement of the area shown in *A*, at the end of the fourth week; *C*, horizontal section of the head of the embryo shown in *A*, showing the floor of the oral cavity and pharynx; *D*, a schematic drawing of the primitive pharynx and its pouches. The laryngotracheal tube and its bronchial buds are also shown; *E* to *J*, successive stages in the development of the tracheoesophageal septum during the fourth week, and separation of the laryngotracheal tube from the esophagus; *E*, *F*, and *G*, lateral views; *H*, *I*, and *J*, transverse sections.

The epithelium of the primitive larynx proliferates rapidly and temporarily occludes its lumen. By the tenth week the excess cells have degenerated and the lumen has been restored. During recanalization, the **laryngeal ventricles** develop which are bounded by *folds of mucous membrane* that become the **vocal folds** (vocal cords) and the **vestibular folds**.

The epiglottis, which serves as *a valve over the inlet of the larynx* (see Fig. 10–2B), develops from the caudal part of the **hypobranchial eminence** (see Figs. 10–1C and 10–2A). This is a median prominence produced by proliferation of mesenchyme in the ventral ends of the third and fourth pairs of branchial arches (see Figs. 10–1C and 10–2A).

The *laryngeal muscles* develop from myoblasts (primitive muscle cells) derived from the fourth and sixth pairs of branchial arches. They are innervated by the laryngeal branches of the vagus nerves that supply these arches (see Table 9–1).

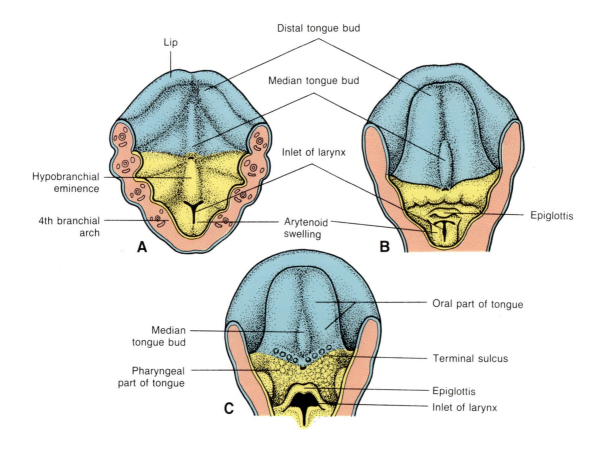

Figure 10–2 Drawings illustrating successive stages in the development of the tongue and larynx between the fourth and tenth week.

Development of the Trachea

The epithelium and glands of the trachea develop from the endoderm of the part of the **laryngotracheal tube** that lies caudal to the developing larynx. The cartilages, connective tissue, and smooth muscle of the trachea are derived from the surrounding splanchnic mesenchyme (see Fig. 10–1G).

Tracheoesophageal Fistula (Fig. 10–3).   This is the most common congenital malformation of the lower respiratory tract. Tracheoesophageal fistula results from *incomplete separation of the trachea and esophagus* during the fourth week (see Fig. 10–1H to J). Tracheoesophageal fistula is commonly associated with **esophageal atresia** (see Fig. 10–3A). There are several varieties of the esophageal atresia and tracheoesophageal fistula malformation. The most common is the one in which the superior part of the esophagus terminates as a blind pouch and its inferior part is joined to the trachea via a fistula (see Fig. 10–3A). Newborn infants with these malformations cough and choke owing to the aspiration of saliva, milk, and gastric contents into the lungs.

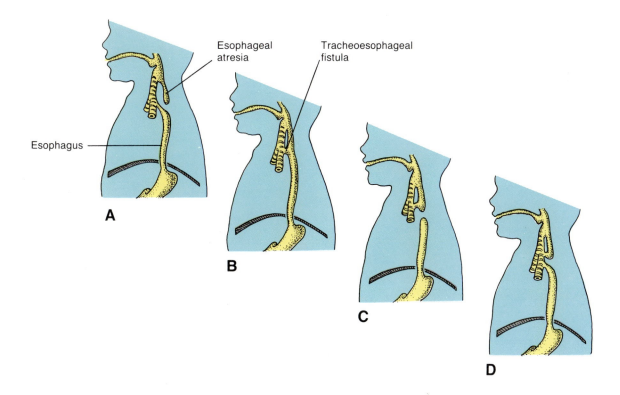

Esophageal atresia

Tracheoesophageal fistula

Esophagus

A

B

C

D

Figure 10–3   Sketches illustrating the common types of tracheoesophageal fistula. The type shown in *A* occurs in about 90 percent of cases. Note that there is also atresia blockage of the esophagus.

Development of the Bronchi

By the end of the fourth week the endodermal lung bud, surrounded by splanchnic mesenchyme, has divided into two **bronchial buds** (see Figs. 10–1G and 10–4A). During the fifth week, each bronchial bud enlarges to form the primordium of a principal or *primary bronchus* (see Fig. 10–4B). From the outset, the embryonic right primary bronchus is slightly larger than the left one and is oriented more vertically (see Fig. 10–4B to E). This embryonic relationship persists throughout life which accounts for the fact that foreign bodies are more likely to enter the right primary bronchus than the left one.

Later in the fifth week, each primary bronchus divides into two more bronchial buds, the primordia of the *secondary bronchi* (see Fig. 10–4C). On *the right*

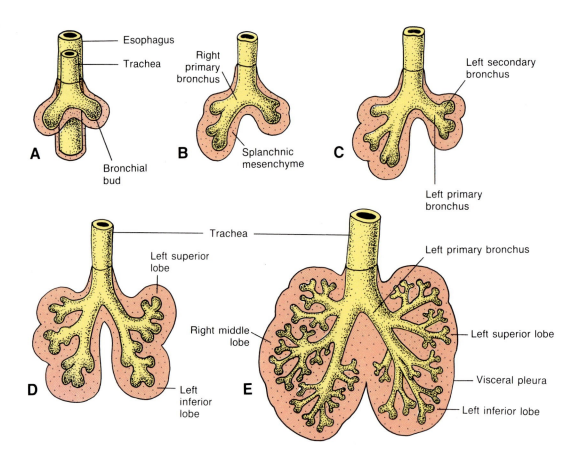

Figure 10–4 Drawings of ventral views of the developing lower respiratory system, showing successive stages in the development of the bronchi and lungs. *A,* 4 weeks; *B* and *C,* 5 weeks; *D,* 6 weeks; *E,* 8 weeks. Note that the splanchnic mesoderm covering the external surface of the lung develops into the visceral pleura (*E*).

side, the superior secondary bronchus supplies the developing superior lobe of the lung. The inferior secondary bronchus redivides to form two bronchi: one supplies the developing middle lobe and the other the developing inferior lobe (see Fig. 10–4C and D). On *the left side*, the two secondary bronchi supply the developing superior and inferior lobes.

Segmental bronchi (tertiary bronchi), ten in the right lung and eight or nine in the left lung, result from the branching of the secondary bronchi during the eighth week (see Fig. 10–4E). Each segmental bronchus, along with its surrounding mesenchyme, is the primordium of a *bronchopulmonary segment* (segment of a lung).

As the bronchi develop, hyaline cartilaginous plates develop in their walls from the surrounding splanchnic mesenchyme. The bronchial smooth musculature and connective tissue and the pulmonary connective tissue and capillaries are also derived from this mesenchyme.

Development of the Lungs

For descriptive purposes, *lung development is divided into four stages or periods:*

1. **The Pseudoglandular Period** (5 to 17 weeks). The developing lung somewhat resembles an exocrine gland during this stage. By 17 weeks, all major parts of the lungs have formed, except those involved with gas exchange. Respiration is not possible during this period; hence, *fetuses born during this initial stage of lung development cannot survive if born prematurely.*

2. **The Canalicular Period** (16 to 25 weeks). During this stage the lumina of the bronchi and terminal bronchioles become larger and highly vascular lung tissue forms (Fig. 10–5A). The terminal bronchioles first divide into several *respiratory bronchioles*, then each respiratory bronchiole gives rise to three to six *alveolar ducts.* Each of these ducts ends in a bulging **terminal sac** (primitive alveolus) that is lined with cuboidal epithelium (see Fig. 10–5A). Some respiration is possible toward the end of the canalicular period because a few terminal sacs have become thin-walled and the tissue around them has become well vascularized (see Fig. 10–5B).

Fetuses born prematurely toward the end of this period (22 to 25 weeks) have a chance of survival if given intensive care, but they often die because their respiratory and other systems are still immature.

3. **The Terminal Sac Period** (24 weeks to birth). Many more terminal sacs (primitive alveoli) develop during this *final prenatal stage.* Between the twenty-fourth and twenty-eighth week, the epithelium lining the terminal sacs becomes so thin that capillaries bulge into them (see Fig. 10–5C). By 24 weeks the terminal sacs are mainly lined by *squamous epithelial cells,* known as *type I pneumocytes.* Scattered amongst these cells are rounded *secretory epithelial cells,* known as *type II pneumocytes.* These specialized alveolar cells secrete *pulmonary surfactant* which lines the interior of the walls of the terminal sacs.

Surfactant counteracts surface tension forces and facilitates expansion of the terminal sacs (primitive alveoli) at birth. Consequently, fetuses born after 24 weeks may survive.

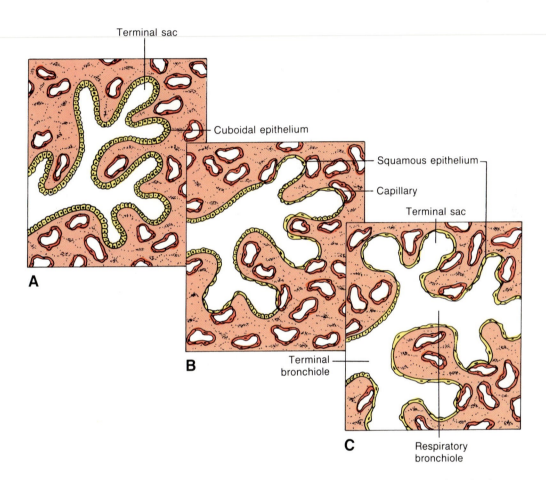

Figure 10–5 Diagrammatic sketches of sections of the lungs, illustrating progressive stages of lung development. *A*, the canalicular period (16 to 25 weeks); *B*, the terminal sac period (24 weeks to birth); *C*, the alveolar period (late fetal period to about 8 years). During the terminal sac period (B), note that the epithelium lining the primitive alveoli (terminal sacs) becomes so thin that the capillaries bulge into them. Respiration becomes possible because the thin squamous epithelium is intimately associated with numerous blood and lymph capillaries.

However, adequate amounts of surfactant are not produced until about the thirty-second week.

Infants born after 32 weeks have a good chance of survival because their lungs are fairly well developed and sufficient surfactant is present. Many alveoli continue to develop during the last six weeks of intrauterine life and for several years after birth.

4. **The Alveolar Period** (late fetal period to about 8 years). At the beginning of this stage, each alveolar duct terminates in a cluster of thin-walled terminal sacs (primitive alveoli) that are separated from each other by loose connective tissue. Before birth, the immature alveoli appear as small bulges from the walls of the alveolar ducts.

Characteristic mature alveoli do not form until some time after birth. Until the third year, enlargement of the lungs results from an increase in the number of immature alveoli rather than from an increase in the size of the alveoli. Thereafter, the number of alveoli continues to increase up to the eighth year, but the size of the alveoli also increases.

The breathing movements that occur before birth result in the aspiration of fluid into the lungs. The lungs at birth are about half filled with fluid derived from the amniotic cavity, tracheal glands, and lungs.

The fluid in the lungs at birth is cleared by three routes: (1) through the mouth and nose; (2) into the pulmonary capillaries; and, (3) into the lymphatics and the pulmonary vessels.

Congenital malformations of the lungs are uncommon. Extra fissures resulting in additional lobes are occasionally observed but these are usually unimportant clinically.

Hypoplasia of the lung(s) occurs in infants with *congenital posterolateral diaphragmatic hernia* (see Fig. 8–3B). The lungs are unable to develop normally and do not expand at birth because they are compressed by the abnormally positioned abdominal viscera (see Chapter 8 and Fig. 8–3).

The respiratory distress syndrome is common in premature infants. It is characterized by rapid, labored breathing. A *deficiency of pulmonary surfactant appears to be the major cause of the respiratory distress associated with* **hyaline membrane disease**. The lungs in these infants are underinflated and a glassy hyaline membrane covers the alveolar surfaces.

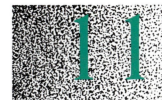

DIGESTIVE SYSTEM

DIGESTIVE SYSTEM

Owing to the formation of the head, tail, and lateral folds during the fourth week (see Fig. 4–1), the dorsal part of the **yolk sac** is incorporated into the embryo as the **primitive gut** (Fig. 11–1A). The primitive gut is the primordium of the digestive system.

The *endoderm* of the primitive gut gives rise to most of the epithelium of the digestive tract and to the parenchyma of its associated glands (e.g., the liver and pancreas). The epithelium at the superior and inferior ends of the digestive tract is derived from the ectoderm of the **stomodeum** (primitive mouth) and **proctodeum** (anal pit), respectively. (see Figs. 11–1 and 11–5).

The connective tissue and muscles in the wall of the digestive tract are derived from the *splanchnic mesenchyme* that surrounds the endodermal primitive gut. For descriptive purposes, the primitive gut is divided into three parts: *foregut*, *midgut*, and *hindgut* (see Fig. 11–1A).

THE FOREGUT

The derivatives of the foregut are: (1) the *pharynx* and its derivatives, which are discussed in Chapter 9 (see page 78); (2) the *lower respiratory system*, described in Chapter 10 (see page 88); (3) the *esophagus*; (4) the *stomach*; (5) the *duodenum*, cranial to the opening of the bile duct; (6) the *liver* and *pancreas*; and (7) the *biliary apparatus* (gallbladder and biliary ducts). All these derivatives, except the pharynx, respiratory tract, and most of the esophagus, are supplied by the *celiac trunk*, the artery of the foregut (see Fig. 11–1A).

Development of the Esophagus

The separation of the esophagus from the laryngotracheal tube by the **tracheoesophageal septum** is described in Chapter 10 and is illustrated in Figure 10–11.

Initially the esophagus is short but it lengthens rapidly, mainly as the result of cranial body growth (especially the growth and descent of the heart and lungs). The esophagus reaches its final relative length by the seventh week. The epithelium and glands of the esophagus are derived from **endoderm**. The striated muscle (skeletal muscle) constituting the muscularis externis, principally in the superior third of the esophagus, is derived from *mesenchyme* in the caudal branchial arches. However the smooth muscle of the esophagus develops from the surrounding splanchnic mesenchyme.

Esophageal Atresia (see Fig. 10–3). Esophageal atresia, usually associated with a *tracheoesophageal fistula*, results from abnormal deviation of the *tracheoesophageal septum* in a posterior direction. As a result, there is incomplete separation of the laryngotracheal tube from the esophagus.

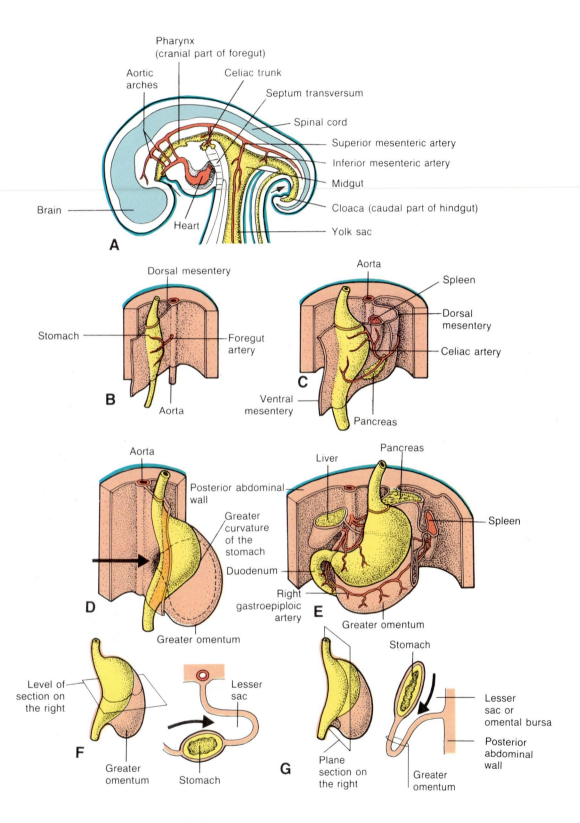

Figure 11–1 Drawings illustrating development of the digestive system. *A,* four weeks; *B,* five weeks; *C,* six weeks; *D* to *F,* seven weeks. The arrow at the cranial (head) end in *A,* indicates the primitive mouth or stomodeum, and the arrow at the caudal (tail) end indicates the anal pit or proctodeum. In *D, F,* and *G,* the arrows indicate the epiploic foramen which is the opening into the lesser sac or omental bursa. The broken line (---) in *D* indicates the location of the lesser sac.

Polyhydramnios (an excessive amount of amniotic fluid) is associated with esophageal atresia because the fetus is unable to swallow amniotic fluid. Hence, amniotic fluid cannot pass to the intestines for absorption and transfer via the placenta to the maternal blood for disposal by the mother's urinary system.

Development of the Stomach

The foregut is a simple tubular structure in the fourth week (see Fig. 11–1A), but a localized dilation of it soon indicates where the stomach is developing (see Fig. 11–1B). The fusiform **primitive stomach**, initially orientated in the median plane, is suspended from the dorsal wall of the abdominal cavity by a **dorsal mesentery** or mesogastrium.

During the fifth and sixth weeks the appearance and position of the stomach change greatly, owing to the different rates of growth of its walls and to enlargement of the liver (see Fig. 11–1E). The primitive stomach enlarges and broadens ventrodorsally and its dorsal border grows faster than its ventral border (see Fig. 11–1C and D). This demarcates the *greater curvature of the stomach*.

Rotation of the Stomach (see Fig. 11–1B to F). As the stomach acquires its characteristic shape, it rotates 90 degrees in a clockwise direction around its longitudinal axis. This causes its left side to face anteriorly and its right side to face posteriorly. Consequently, the left vagus nerve that initially innervated the left side of the stomach now innervates the anterior wall. Similarly, the right vagus nerve comes to innervate the posterior wall of the stomach.

Mesenteries of the Stomach (see Figs. 11–1 and 11–2). The dorsal mesentery of the stomach, often called the **dorsal mesogastrium**, suspends the stomach from the dorsal wall of the abdominal cavity and a ventral mesentery or **ventral mesogastrium** attaches the stomach and the cranial part of duodenum to the liver and the ventral abdominal wall. After rotation and growth of the stomach, the part of the dorsal mesentery that is attached to its greater curvature hangs caudally as a pouch-like fold of peritoneum, known as the *greater omentum* (see Fig. 11–1E).

Formation of the Omental Bursa. Rotation of the stomach also results in formation of the *omental bursa* or lesser peritoneal sac (lesser sac), a recess of the peritoneal cavity that is located posterior to the stomach (see Fig. 11–1E and F). As the stomach enlarges, the omental bursa expands and acquires an *inferior recess* between the layers of the greater omentum (see Fig. 11–1F and G). This recess almost completely disappears as the layers of the greater omentum fuse (Fig. 11–4B and D). The **lesser sac of peritoneum** or omental bursa communicates with the main part of the peritoneal cavity or *greater sac of peritoneum* through an opening called the *epiploic foramen* or foramen of Winslow (see Fig. 11–1F and G).

Congenital Hypertrophic Pyloric Stenosis. In about one in every 150 male and in one in 750 female infants, there is a *marked thickening of the pyloric region of the stomach*. This hypertrophy involves the circular, and, to a lesser degree, the longitudinal muscle fibers of the **pylorus**. Associated with pyloric stenosis there is a *severe narrowing* (G. *stenosis*, a narrowing) of the pyloric canal and obstruction to the passage of food into the duodenum. As a result, the infant expels the contents of the stomach with considerable force (*projectile vomiting*).

Development of the Duodenum

The epithelium of the duodenum and the parenchyma (epithelial elements) of the accessory glands (e.g., pancreas) of this first part of the small intestine are derived from the caudal part of the foregut and the cranial part of the midgut (Fig. 11-2B and D). Other parts of its wall arise from the adjacent mesenchyme. The junction of the two embryonic parts of the duodenum is located just distal to the origin of the bile duct (common bile duct). As the stomach rotates, the duodenum develops a C-shaped loop and rotates to the right, where it comes to lie retroperitoneally (external to the peritoneum).

Because of its origin from both the foregut and midgut, the duodenum is supplied by branches of the celiac trunk (foregut artery) and the superior mesenteric artery (midgut artery).

During the fifth and sixth weeks, the lumen of the duodenum becomes partly or wholly occluded owing to the proliferation of its lining of epithelial cells. Normally, the duodenum is recanalized by the end of the eighth week.

Partial or complete failure of this process results in either **duodenal stenosis** (narrowing) or **duodenal atresia** (blockage). The descending, or second, part of the duodenum is most commonly involved, usually just distal to the *hepatopancreatic ampulla*, the dilation that normally receives both the bile duct and the main pancreatic duct.

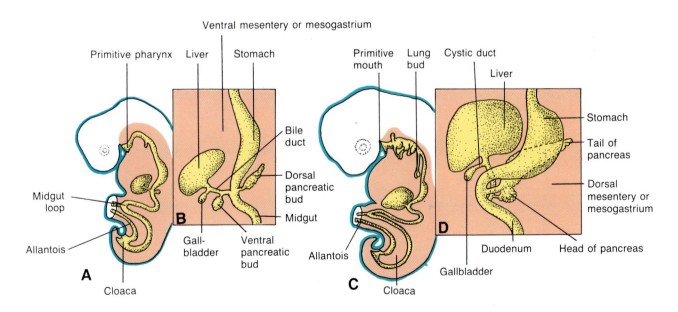

Figure 11-2 Drawings illustrating successive stages in the development of the duodenum, liver, pancreas, and extrahepatic biliary apparatus during the fourth to sixth week. The duodenum develops from the caudal part of the foregut (distal to the stomach) and the cranial part of the midgut (distal to the entrance of the pancreatic duct).

Development of the Pancreas

The pancreas develops from two outgrowths of the endodermal epithelium lining the caudal part of the foregut. These outgrowths, known as the **ventral pancreatic bud** and the **dorsal pancreatic bud**, are located on the ventral and dorsal aspects of the foregut, respectively (see Fig. 11-2B). Owing to rotation and differential growth of the foregut, the ventral pancreatic bud and bile duct migrate dorsally around the duodenum. Here *the ventral pancreatic bud fuses with the dorsal pancreatic bud* (see Fig. 11-2D). The ducts of the two pancreatic buds join and the combined duct becomes the *main pancreatic duct* that opens with the bile duct into the duodenum. The proximal part of the duct of the dorsal pancreatic bud may persist as an *accessory pancreatic duct* which opens into the duodenum cranial to the main duct. The ventral pancreatic bud forms most of the head of the pancreas; the dorsal pancreatic bud forms the remainder of the pancreas (i.e., the body and tail).

Development of the Spleen

This lymphatic organ develops from a mass of mesenchymal cells located between the layers of the dorsal mesentery of the stomach (see Fig. 11-1C and E). The spleen is lobulated in the fetus, but the lobules normally disappear before birth. The notches in the superior border of the adult spleen are remnants of the grooves that separated the fetal lobules.

Development of the Liver and Biliary Apparatus

The liver, gallbladder, and biliary ducts arise as a ventral outgrowth of the endodermal epithelium from the caudal part of the foregut early in the fourth week (see Fig. 11-2A and B). This **hepatic diverticulum** (*liver bud*), consists of rapidly proliferating endodermal cell strands that *extend into the septum transversum*. The **septum transversum** is a mass of mesoderm between the pericardial cavity and the yolk stalk (see Fig. 11-1A). The septum transversum forms a major part of the diaphragm (see Fig. 8-2B), and in this region it also forms the ventral mesentery (see Fig. 11-1C).

As the hepatic diverticulum grows, it enlarges rapidly and divides into two parts. The large **cranial part** is the primordium of the parenchyma of the liver. The hemopoietic cells, Kupfer cells, and connective tissue cells are derived from mesenchyme in the septum transversum. The small **caudal part** gives rise to the *gallbladder* and *cystic duct* (see Fig. 11-2D). The liver grows rapidly and intermingles with the vitelline and umbilical veins. The liver soon fills most of the abdominal cavity.

Hemopoiesis (blood formation) begins during the *sixth week*. This activity is mainly responsible for the relatively large size of the liver between the seventh and ninth weeks of development. *Bile formation* by the hepatic cells begins during the *twelfth week*.

Extrahepatic Biliary Atresia.   Blockage of the bile ducts results from their failure to recanalize following the solid stage of their development. This severe malformation could also result from interference with the blood supply of the ducts resulting from liver infection during the fetal period.

THE MIDGUT

The derivatives of the midgut are: (1) the *small intestine*, including most of the duodenum; (2) the *cecum* and *vermiform appendix*; (3) the *ascending colon*; and, (4) *most of the transverse colon*. All these midgut derivatives are supplied by the **superior mesenteric artery**, the artery of the midgut (see Figs. 11–1A and 11–3A).

The midgut is suspended from the abdominal wall by an elongated dorsal mesentery (see Fig. 11–3A). It communicates with the yolk sac via the **yolk stalk**.

Formation and Herniation of the Midgut Loop.   As the midgut lengthens, it forms a ventral U-shaped loop, called the midgut loop, which projects into the remains of the extraembryonic coelom in the proximal part of the umbilical cord (see Fig. 11–2). This herniation, often referred to as a **physiological umbilical herniation**, is a normal passage of the midgut into the umbilical cord. The midgut loop has *cranial and caudal limbs*. The caudal limb is easily recognized because of the **cecal diverticulum** on its antimesenteric aspect (see Fig. 11–3B). The *cranial limb* lengthens rapidly, forming *loops of small intestine*, but the caudal limb undergoes very little change.

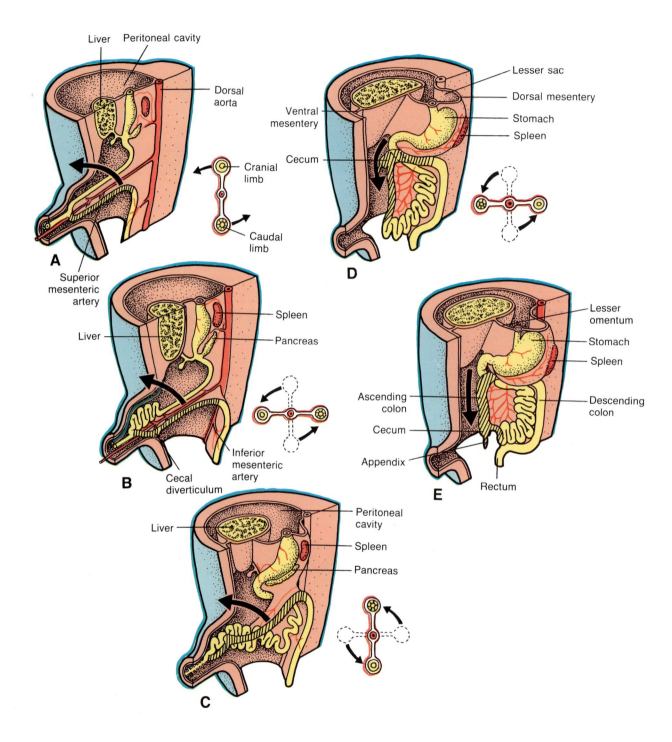

Figure 11–3 Drawings showing development and rotation of the midgut from the sixth to the eleventh week. During rotation, the midgut elongates and coils to form loops of small bowel. It also forms a large part of the large bowel (see striped areas such as ascending colon in *E*).

Rotation of the Midgut Loop   (see Fig. 11–3B to E). While in the umbilical cord, *the midgut loop rotates 90 degrees counterclockwise around an axis formed by the superior mesenteric artery.* This brings the cranial limb of the midgut loop to the right and the caudal limb to the left (see Fig. 11–3B). During the tenth week the intestines rapidly return to the abdomen, a process that is sometimes called *the reduction of the midgut hernia.* The small intestine returns first, passing posterior to the superior mesenteric artery and occupying the central part of the abdomen. The cecum, being the widest part of the intestine, returns last. It occupies the right side of the abdomen (see Fig. 11–3D), just caudal to the right lobe of the liver, which extends to the lower lumbar region at this stage. As the intestines return to the abdominal cavity, they undergo a further 180-degree counterclockwise rotation, making a total of 270 degrees (see Fig. 11–3C and D). The ascending colon becomes recognizable as the posterior abdominal wall elongates (see Fig. 11–3E).

Fixation of the Intestines   (Fig. 11–4). The attachment of the dorsal mesentery to the posterior abdominal wall is greatly modified after the intestines return to the abdominal cavity. As the intestines enlarge, lengthen, and assume their final positions, their mesenteries are pressed against the posterior abdominal wall. Initially the mesentery of the small intestine is continuous

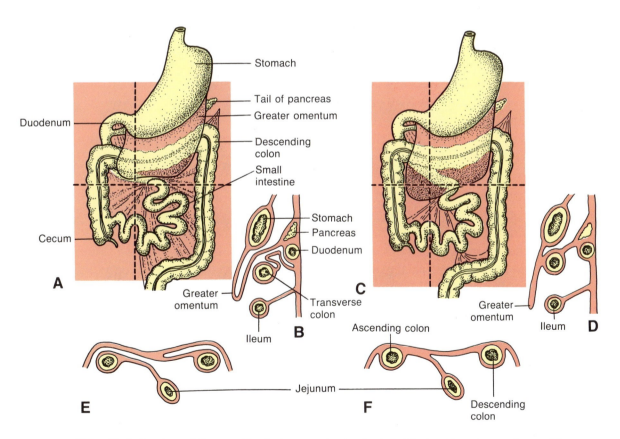

Figure 11–4   Drawings of the gastrointestinal system, showing fixation of the intestines. *A,* ventral view of the intestines prior to their fixation; *B,* sagittal section at the plane shown in *A,* showing the greater omentum overhanging the transverse colon; *C,* ventral view of the intestines after their fixation; *D,* sagittal section at the plane shown in *C; E,* transverse section at the level shown in *A; F,* transverse section at the level shown in *C.*

with that of the transverse mesocolon. The mesentery of the ascending and descending colon fuses with the parietal peritoneum on this wall and disappears. As a result, *the ascending and descending colon become retroperitoneal*, i.e., external to the peritoneum (see Fig. 11-4E and F).

The colon presses the duodenum against the posterior abdominal wall. As a result, most of the duodenal mesentery is absorbed and almost all of the duodenum becomes retroperitoneal, as does most of the pancreas (see Fig. 11-4B and D). As this occurs, the small intestines acquire a new line of attachment that extends from where the duodenum becomes retroperitoneal to the ileocecal junction (see Fig. 11-4C). The mesentery of the transverse colon fuses with the dorsal mesogastrium to form the posterior wall of the inferior part of the omental bursa. The sigmoid colon (pelvic colon) retains its mesentery, but it is shorter than in the early fetus (see Fig. 11-4C).

The Cecum and Vermiform Appendix. The primordium of the cecum and appendix, called the *cecal diverticulum*, appears during the sixth week as a swelling on the antimesenteric border of the cranial part of the caudal limb of the midgut loop (see Fig. 11-3B). The apex of the cecal diverticulum does not grow as rapidly as the rest; as a result, the appendix forms (see Fig. 11-3E). After birth, the wall of the cecum grows unequally, causing the appendix to become located on the medial side of the cecum. It usually lies retrocecally.

The appendix is relatively long at birth but becomes shorter during childhood.

Malformations of the Midgut

Ileal Diverticulum (Meckel's Diverticulum). This is the most common malformation of the midgut. A Meckel's diverticulum *is a remnant of the proximal part of the yolk stalk* which fails to degenerate and disappear during the early fetal period. It is usually a finger-like blind sac, about 5 cm long, that projects from the antimesenteric border of the ileum. In adults it is usually located 40 to 50 cm from the ileocecal junction. A Meckel's diverticulum occurs in about two percent of people. It usually remains symptomless, but rectal bleeding, with or without abdominal pain, may occur.

Omphalocele. This condition results when the midgut fails to return to the abdominal cavity from the umbilical cord during the tenth week. Coils of intestine protrude from the umbilicus and are covered by a transparent sac of amnion.

Malrotations of the Midgut. Various malformations of the intestines result when the midgut does not rotate normally as it returns to the abdominal cavity from the umbilical cord. An infant with malrotation usually *presents with symptoms of intestinal obstruction* shortly after birth. Often this is caused by a peritoneal band that runs from an abnormally positioned cecum to the right side of the abdomen, crossing the descending part of the duodenum. Malrotation also predisposes to a **volvulus of the midgut** where there is a twisting of the intestines around a short mesentery. Usually volvulus interferes with the blood supply to the intestines.

Subhepatic Cecum and Appendix. If the cecum and appendix adhere to the inferior surface of the liver during the early fetal period, they will be carried superiorly as the liver diminishes in size. As a result, the cecum and appendix are located in the fetal position shown in Figure 11–3D. This condition, more common in males than in females, occurs in about six percent of fetuses. A subhepatic cecum and appendix are not common in adults. However, when the condition exists it may create a diagnostic problem in *appendicitis* and during removal of the appendix (*appendectomy*).

Stenosis and Atresia of the Small Intestine.   Narrowing (stenosis) and complete obstruction (atresia) of the intestines occur most often in the duodenum and ileum. Most of these malformations result from the failure of recanalization to occur following the solid stage of intestinal development. Some stenoses and atresias of the ileum may be caused by an infarction of the fetal bowel owing to impairment of its blood supply. This would most likely result from a volvulus of the intestines that forms as they return from the umbilical cord.

THE HINDGUT

Hindgut Derivatives.   The derivatives of the hindgut are: (1) the *left part of the transverse colon*; (2) the *descending colon*; (3) the *sigmoid colon*; (4) the *rectum*; (5) the *superior portion of the anal canal*; and, (6) the epithelium of the urinary bladder and most of the urethra (see Fig. 11–5E). All these derivatives are supplied by the *inferior mesenteric artery*, the artery of the hindgut (see Fig. 11–1A). The junction between the part of the transverse colon derived from the midgut and the part derived from the hindgut is indicated by the change in blood supply. The former is supplied by a branch of the *superior mesenteric artery* (midgut artery) and the latter by a branch of the *inferior mesenteric artery* (hindgut artery).

Partitioning of the Cloaca (Fig. 11–5).   The caudal part of the hindgut expands into the **cloaca**, an endodermal-lined cavity that is in contact with the surface ectoderm at the **cloacal membrane** (see Fig. 11–5A). The cloacal membrane lies at the bottom of a depression known as the **proctodeum** or anal pit (see Fig. 11–5B). The cloaca is divided into dorsal and ventral parts by a coronal sheet of mesenchyme, called the **urorectal septum** (see Fig. 11–5A), that *develops in the angle between the allantois and the hindgut* (see Fig. 11–5B).

The urorectal septum slowly grows caudally, dividing the cloaca into a ventral portion, called the primitive **urogenital sinus**, and a dorsal portion, often referred to as the **anorectal canal**, because it develops into part of the rectum and the anal canal (see Fig. 11–5C). By seven weeks, the urorectal septum reaches the cloacal membrane and divides it into a ventral **urogenital membrane** and a dorsal **anal membrane**. The area of fusion of the urorectal septum with the cloacal membrane is represented by the *central perineal tendon* (perineal body). The central perineal tendon is the center and *landmark of the perineum*, where several muscles converge and insert into it.

The Anal Canal

The epithelium of the superior two thirds of the anal canal is derived from the endodermal **hindgut**; the inferior one third develops from the ectodermal **proctodeum** (see Fig. 11–5B and C). The junction of the epithelium derived from the endoderm of the hindgut and the ectoderm of the proctodeum is indicated by the irregular *pectinate line*, located at the inferior limit of the *anal valves*. This line also indicates the approximate former site of the anal membrane (see Fig. 11–5C) that ruptures in the eighth week. The other layers of the wall of the anal canal are derived from the surrounding splanchnic mesenchyme.

The dual origin of the anal canal is indicated by its blood supply, venous and lymphatic drainage, and nerve supply. The superior two thirds of the anal canal are mainly supplied by the *superior rectal artery*, the continuation of the *inferior mesenteric artery* (the hindgut artery). The venous drainage of this part is mainly by the *superior rectal veins*, tributaries of the *inferior mesenteric vein*. The lymphatic drainage of the superior two thirds of the anal canal is eventually to the *inferior mesenteric lymph nodes*.

The inferior third of the anal canal, which is derived from the ectodermal proctodeum, is supplied mainly by the *inferior rectal arteries*, branches of the *internal pudendal arteries*. The venous drainage of this inferior part is by the *inferior rectal veins*, tributaries of the *internal pudendal veins*, that drain into the internal iliac veins. The lymphatic drainage of this part of the canal is to the *superficial inguinal lymph nodes*.

The nerve supply of the superior two thirds of the anal canal is via the *autonomic nervous system*, whereas the inferior third is supplied by the *inferior rectal nerve* via the *sacral plexus*.

The above-mentioned differences in blood supply, venous and lymphatic drainage, and nerve supply of the anal canal are important clinically, e.g., when considering the spread of tumors.

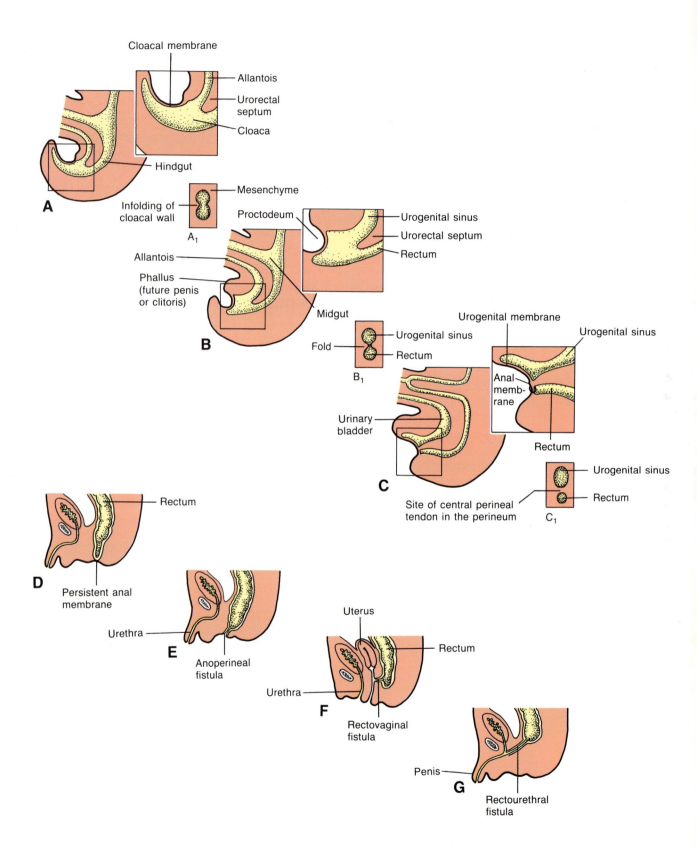

Figure 11-5 Drawings illustrating successive stages in the partitioning of the cloaca into the rectum and urogenital sinus between the fourth and seventh weeks.

Anorectal Malformations

Malformations of the anal canal and rectum constitute the largest group of congenital abnormalities of the digestive tract. *Anorectal malformations result from abnormal growth and development of the urorectal septum* (see Fig. 11–5D to G). These malformations are usually classified clinically into two groups: high and low anorectal malformations, depending on whether the rectum terminates superior or inferior to the *puborectal sling,* a muscular band of the puborectalis muscle that *passes around the anorectal junction.*

High Anorectal Malformations (See Fig. 11–5F and G).   These malformations account for most congenital abnormalities of the anorectal region and are commonly associated with **fistulas** (L. *fistulae,* pipes or tubes). The rectum ends as a blind pouch superior to the puborectal sling. In males, the fistulas or *abnormal passages* connect anteriorly with the urinary bladder (**rectovesical fistula**) or the urethra (**rectourethral fistula**). In females, the fistulas connect anteriorly with the vagina (**rectovaginal fistula**) or the vestible of the vagina (**rectovestibular fistula**).

Low Anorectal Malformations (See Fig. 11–5D and E).   These malformations result from failure of the anal membrane to rupture in the eighth week. As a result, *the embryonic proctodeum (anal pit) persists* and does not communicate with the part of the anal canal derived from the hindgut. This malformation is usually referred to as **imperforate anus.** In simple cases, the urorectal septum has developed normally and the anal canal is separated from the exterior by a thin covering of skin (see Fig. 11–5D). In other cases, there are fistulous communications with the perineum (see Fig. 11–5E). The abnormal opening of the fistula is sometimes referred to as an *"ectopic anus."*

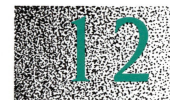

UROGENITAL SYSTEM

UROGENITAL SYSTEM

Embryologically and functionally, the urogenital system can be divided into two parts: (1) *the urinary system* and (2) *the genital system*. Both systems develop from the **intermediate mesoderm** (Fig. 12–1A) and the excretory ducts of both systems initially enter a common cavity called the **cloaca** (Fig. 12–2A).

As development proceeds, the overlapping of the two systems is particularly obvious in the male. The primitive excretory duct of the mesonephric kidney, called the **mesonephric duct**, (see Fig. 12–2A$_1$) serves originally as a urinary duct. Later, the mesonephric duct is transformed into the main genital duct (Fig. 12–3C), the *ductus deferens* (vas deferens).

The *ureter* develops from an outgrowth of the caudal end of the mesonephric duct, known as the **metanephric diverticulum** or ureteric bud (see Fig. 12–2A). In the adult male, the urinary and genital organs discharge their excretions, urine and semen respectively, through a common urogenital canal in the penis, known as the *spongy urethra* (see Fig. 12–3C).

When the embryo folds in the horizontal plane during the fourth week, the intermediate mesoderm is carried ventrally where it loses its connection with the somites (see Fig. 12–1). After folding, the intermediate mesoderm forms a longitudinal mass on each side of the primitive aorta in the trunk region, called the **urogenital ridge** (see Fig. 12–1C). The urinary and genital systems develop from the mesoderm in these ridges. The part of the urogenital ridge that gives rise to the urinary system is known as the **nephrogenic cord** (see Fig. 12–1C) or *nephrogenic ridge*, and the part that gives rise to the genital system is known as the **gonadal ridge** or *genital ridge* (Fig. 12–4A). Development of the urinary system begins first.

THE URINARY SYSTEM

Development of the Kidneys

Three different sets of kidneys develop in human embryos (see Fig. 12–2A): the **pronephros, mesonephros,** and **metanephros** (the permanent kidney).

The first pair of "kidneys", called pronephroi (plural of pronephros), are rudimentary and nonfunctional (see Fig. 12–2A). The second pair of kidneys or mesonephroi function for a short time during the early fetal period and degenerate as they are replaced by the metanephroi or permanent kidneys (see Fig. 12–2A$_1$).

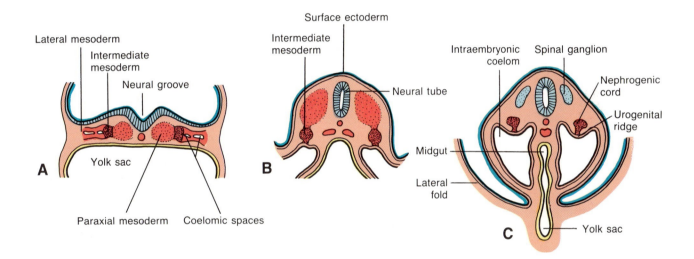

Figure 12–1 Transverse sections of embryos during the fourth week, showing the change in position of the intermediate mesoderm that occurs as the result of folding of the embryo in the transverse plane. In *C*, observe that the intermediate mesoderm forms longitudinal nephrogenic cords that produce bulges of the coelomic epithelium; these are called urogenital ridges.

The Metanephros or Permanent Kidney (See Fig. 12–2). The permanent kidneys begin to develop in the early part of the fifth week while the mesonephroi are still developing. Urine formation begins toward the end of the first trimester (11 to 12 weeks) and continues actively throughout fetal life. Urine is excreted into the amniotic cavity and forms a major part of the amniotic fluid. Because the placenta eliminates metabolic wastes from the fetal blood, there is no need for the kidneys to function before birth; however, they must be able to assume their excretory and regulatory roles at birth.

The permanent kidneys or metanephroi develop from two different sources: (1) the **metanephric diverticulum** or *ureteric bud* and (2) the **metanephric mesoderm** (see Fig. 12–2B). Both primordia are mesodermal derivatives. The metanephric mesoderm is derived from the caudal part of the nephrogenic cord or ridge, and the metanephric diverticulum is a dorsal outgrowth from the mesonephric duct near its entrance into the cloaca (see Fig. 12–2A and B).

The **ureteric bud** or metanephric diverticulum gives rise to the *ureter, renal pelvis, calyces,* and *collecting tubules* (see Fig. 12–2C to E). The **metanephric diverticulum** penetrates the metanephric mesoderm and induces the formation of a *metanephric cap of mesoderm* over its expanded end. Each collecting tubule derived from this diverticulum or ureteric bud undergoes repeated branching to form successive generations of collecting tubules. The first three to four generations of tubules enlarge and become confluent to form the *major calyces* and the second four generations of tubules coalesce to form the *minor calyces* (see Fig. 12–2D). The remaining generations of tubules form the collecting tubules of the permanent kidney.

The ends of the arched collecting tubules induce clusters of mesenchymal cells in the metanephric mesoderm to form **metanephric vesicles** (see Fig. 12–2E and F). These vesicles soon grow and become **metanephric tubules** (see Fig. 12–2H). As these tubules develop, their proximal ends are invaginated by *glomeruli* (plexuses of capillaries). The *renal corpuscle* (glomerulus and Bowman's capsule) and its proximal convoluted tubule, loop of Henle, and distal convoluted tubule constitute a **nephron** (see Fig. 12–2I). Each distal convoluted tubule contacts an arched collecting tubule and then the tubules become confluent, forming a *uriniferous tubule.* Consequently, *each uriniferous tubule consists of two embryologically different parts:* a nephron, derived from metanephric mesoderm, and a collecting tubule, derived from the metanephric diverticulum (see Fig. 12–2).

Positional Changes and Blood Supply of the Developing Kidneys. Initially the kidneys lie close together in the pelvis. As the abdomen grows, the kidneys gradually come to lie in the abdomen and are separated from each other. They normally attain their adult position by the ninth week. This migration or relative ascent results mainly from growth of the embryo caudal to the kidneys. As the kidneys "ascend" from the pelvis, they are supplied by arteries from the aorta at successively higher levels. Normally, the caudal vessels disappear as the kidneys "ascend", but some of them may persist. This accounts for the relatively common variations in the blood supply to the kidneys. About 25 percent of adult kidneys have two to four renal arteries.

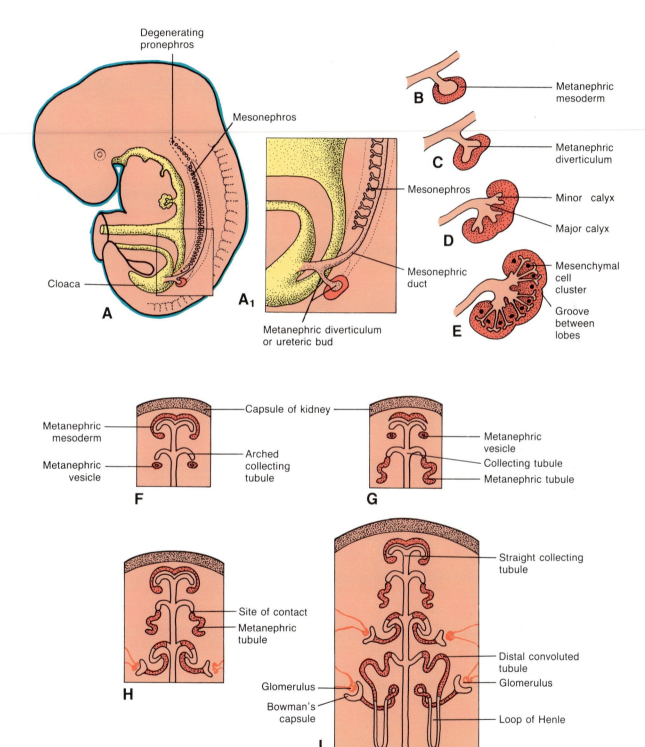

Figure 12–2 *A*, sketch of a lateral view of a five-week embryo, showing the three sets of kidneys that develop in the embryo. The pronephros is rudimentary and nonfunctional. The mesonephros functions for about two weeks and then degenerates. The metanephros develops into the permanent kidney. *B* to *E*, are sketches of the developing metanephric kidney during the fifth to eighth weeks. *F* to *I*, are diagrammatic sketches illustrating the stages in the development of a nephron. This process begins in the eighth week, but the kidneys do not start to function until 11 to 12 weeks. (Modified from Moore KL. The developing human. Clinically oriented embryology. 4th ed. Philadelphia: WB Saunders, 1988.)

The Fetal and Newborn Kidneys.   The kidneys are subdivided into lobes that are visible externally as elevations that are separated by grooves. This lobation diminishes by the end of the fetal period, but the lobes are still indicated externally in the kidneys of a newborn infant. In adults, the lobated character of the kidneys is usually obscured.

Congenital Malformations of the Kidneys.   Absence of the kidneys (*bilateral renal agenesis*) results when the metanephric diverticula or ureteric buds fail to develop, or when they degenerate before they can induce the metanephric mesoderm to form nephrons. Because the uriniferous tubules develop from two different sources, the failure of the tubules to join, as illustrated in Figure 12–2 G to I, results in **congenital polycystic disease of the kidneys.**

Division of the ureteric bud at an early stage results in a **divided kidney** or a **double kidney.** These abnormal kidneys often have *ectopic ureters* that open into the urethra in males and into the urethra or vagina in females. Abnormal positions of the kidney, such as **pelvic kidney**, result from failure of the kidneys to "ascend" from the pelvis to the abdomen. A **horseshoe kidney** forms when the inferior poles of the kidney fuse while they are in the pelvis.

Development of the Urinary Bladder

The urinary bladder is derived from the hindgut derivative known as the **urogenital sinus** (Fig. 12–3A). It is an endodermal-lined cavity that is formed when the **urorectal septum** divides the cloaca into a dorsal rectum and a ventral urogenital sinus (Fig. 12–3A to C). The caudal ends of the mesonephric ducts open into the cloaca (see Fig. 12–3B) and parts of them are gradually absorbed into the wall of the urinary bladder (see Fig. 12–3E to H). Consequently, the ureters, derived from the metanephric diverticula (ureteric buds), and the mesonephric ducts eventually enter the bladder separately (see Fig. 12–3H).

Owing to the "ascent" of the kidneys, the orifices of the ureters move cranially and the **primordia of the ejaculatory ducts**, derived from the distal ends of the mesonephric ducts, move toward each other and enter the *prostatic part of the urethra* (see Fig. 12–3 G and H).

Although the epithelium of the **trigone** region of the bladder and the cranial part of the prostatic urethra are initially mesodermal in origin, this epithelium is eventually replaced by endodermal cells from the urogenital sinus. Consequently, the epithelium of the urinary bladder and most of the urethra is lined with epithelium of endodermal origin. The surrounding *connective tissue* and *smooth muscle* are derived from the adjacent **splanchnic mesoderm.**

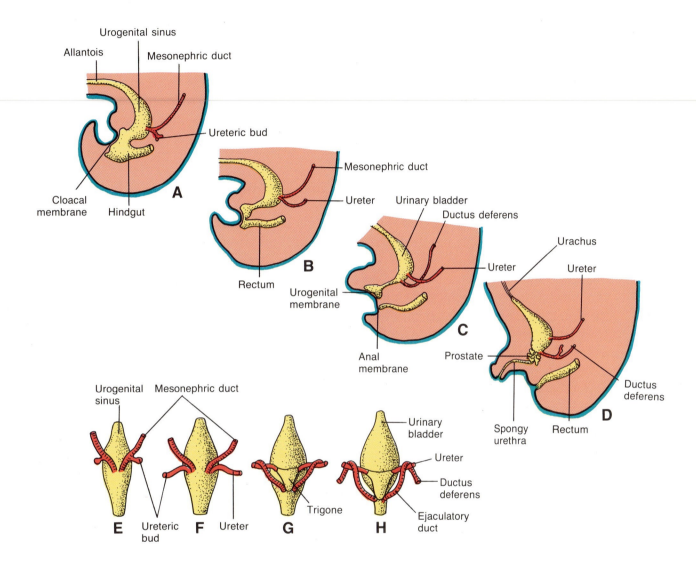

Figure 12-3 Drawings of embryos between the fifth and eighth weeks, showing how the cloaca is divided by the urorectal septum into the urogenital sinus and rectum. Also shown is the relationship of the developing ureters to the mesonephric ducts. The ureter develops as an outgrowth of the mesonephric duct, but it gradually acquires a separate opening into the urinary bladder as the mesonephric duct is absorbed by the bladder. The trigone region of the urinary bladder is formed by the incorporation of the mesonephric ducts. As the kidneys "ascend" from the pelvis, the orifices of the ureters move further cranially (superiorly).

Exstrophy of the Bladder.   This malformation is characterized by the exposure and protrusion of the posterior wall of the urinary bladder which contains the trigone of the bladder and the ureteric orifices. *Exstrophy of the bladder is caused by the defective closure of the inferior part of the anterior abdominal wall.* The fissure involves the anterior abdominal wall and the anterior wall of the urinary bladder. The posterior wall of the bladder protrudes through the defect in the abdominal wall. This severe defect results from the failure of mesenchyme to migrate between the surface ectoderm and the endoderm of the urogenital sinus during the fourth week. As a result, no muscle or connective tissue forms in the anterior abdominal wall over the urinary bladder. The thin epidermis and the anterior wall of the bladder soon rupture.

Development of the Urethra

The epithelium of the female urethra and most of the epithelium of the male urethra is derived from the endoderm of the urogenital sinus (see Fig. 12–3D). The surrounding connective and smooth muscle tissue are derived from the adjacent splanchnic mesoderm. The epithelium of the spongy urethra in the male has a dual origin. Most of it is derived from the endoderm of the urogenital sinus, but the distal portion of the urethra lining the navicular fossa is derived from the surface ectoderm (Fig. 12–5A).

Development of the Prostate Gland

This *auxiliary genital gland* is derived from evaginations, or buds, of the epithelium of the prostatic portion of the urethra which penetrate the surrounding mesenchyme. Consequently, the parenchyma, which includes both the secretory units and ducts, is derived from endoderm, while the smooth muscle and supporting connective tissue are derived from the adjacent splanchnic mesoderm. The urethral and paraurethral glands in the female are homologous to the prostate gland.

The Urachus

Initially the urinary bladder is continuous with the **allantois** (see Fig. 12–3A). The allantois may make a small contribution to the apex of the bladder, but most of it regresses and becomes a fibrous cord, known as the **urachus** (see Fig. 12–3D). This ligament passes from the apex of the bladder to the umbilicus. Occasionally, the lumen of the allantois persists as the urachus forms. This may give rise to a **urachal fistula**, from which urine may drain from the bladder to the exterior via the umbilicus. If only a small part of the lumen of the allantois persists, it may give rise to a **urachal cyst.** If a larger portion of the lumen of the urachus persists, it may give rise to a **urachal sinus** that may open at the umbilicus or into the urinary bladder.

THE GENITAL SYSTEM

Although the genetic sex (chromosomal sex) of an embryo is determined at fertilization by the kind of sperm that fertilizes the ovum (Chapter 1), there are no morphologic indications of maleness or femaleness until the seventh week. The initial period of genital development is called the *indifferent stage of the reproductive organs* because the early genital system is similar in both sexes.

Development of the Gonads (Ovaries and Testes)

The gonads are the first parts of the genital system to undergo development. The primitive gonads are derived from the parts of the urogenital ridges (see Fig. 12-1C) known as the genital or **gonadal ridges** (see Fig. 12-4A). The gonads in both sexes are initially similar and appear as thickenings of the coelomic epithelium (mesothelium lining the peritoneal cavity). Each genital ridge enlarges and frees itself from the mesonephros by developing a mesentery, which becomes the *mesorchium* in the male (see Fig. 12-4B) and the *mesovarium* in the female (see Fig. 12-4E). As this occurs, the coelomic epithelium covering the primitive gonads proliferates and forms cords of cells, called **primary sex cords**, that grow into the mesenchyme of the developing gonads (see Fig. 12-4A).

The primordial germ cells orginate in the wall of the yolk sac and migrate into the embryo and enter the primary sex cords (see Fig. 12-4A). They eventually give rise to the ova and sperms.

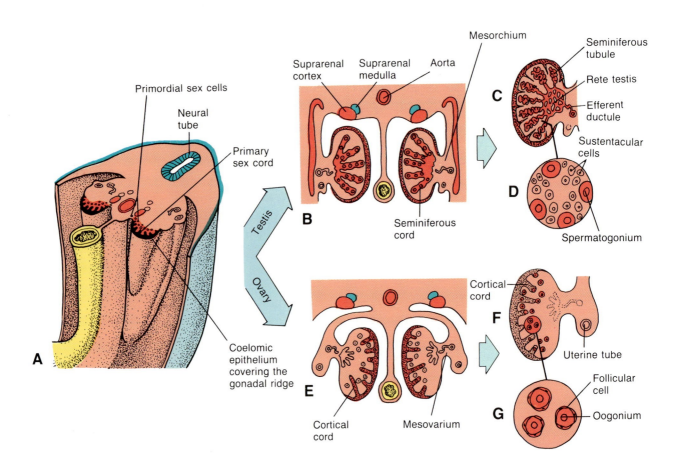

Figure 12–4 *A*, three-dimensional sketch of the caudal region of a five-week embryo, showing the gonadal ridges. Note the primordial sex cells that are migrating from the yolk sac to the gonads; *B*, drawing of the testes at seven weeks, showing the seminiferous cords; *C*, drawing of the testes at 20 weeks, showing the seminiferous tubules; *D*, section of a seminiferous tubule. Note that no lumen is present at this stage and that there are two kinds of cell: sustentacular cells (of Sertoli) and spermatogonia, which comprise the primordia of the sperms; *E*, ovary at 20 weeks, showing the cortical cords and primordial follicles; and *G*, enlarged drawing of three primordial follicles. (Modified from Moore KL. The developing human. Clinically oriented embryology. 4th ed. Philadelphia: WB Saunders 1988.)

The Development of Testes (See Fig. 12–4B, C, and D).   In embryos with a Y chromosome, the primary sex cords, containing primordial germ cells, are soon cut off from the surface epithelium by a dense connective tissue layer, known as the *tunica albuginea*. Septa grow deeply from the tunica albuginea that divide the testes into compartments.

The primary sex cords differentiate into **seminiferous cords** (see Fig. 12–4B) which later become canalized to form *seminiferous tubules*. Within the seminiferous cords, the **primordial germ cells** differentiate into *spermatogonia*, the precursors of sperms (see Fig. 12–4D). The remaining cells in these cords become *sustentacular cells* (*Sertoli cells*). Groups of *interstitial cells* differentiate from the mesenchyme between the developing seminiferous tubules. These cells begin to secrete *testosterone* and other substances before the end of the embryonic period. These hormones are responsible for the differentiation of male genital ducts and external genitalia.

The differentiation of indifferent gonads into testes is largely dependent upon the action of the H-Y androgen on the Y chromosome. The central ends of the developing seminiferous tubules converge and fuse to form a network of canals called the *rete testis* (see Fig. 12–4C). The rete testis connects with several persisting mesonephric tubules which become the *efferent ductules* of the testes.

The Development of Ovaries (See Fig. 12–4E, F, and G).   In embryos lacking a Y chromosome, differentiation of the gonads occurs later than in males. The primary sex cords converge to form a network of canals called the *rete ovarii* which soon disappears along with the primary sex cords. As this occurs, the surface epithelium of the developing ovary gives rise to **secondary sex cords**, or **cortical cords** (see Fig. 12–4E). As these cords grow in the ovary, primordial germ cells are incorporated into them. At about 16 weeks, the cortical cords break up into isolated cell clusters called *primordial follicles* (see Fig. 12–4F), each of which contains an *oogonium* derived from the primordial germ cell. Each oogonium is surrounded by a layer of flattened follicular cells derived from the surface epithelial cells in the cortical cord (see Fig. 12–4G). The oogonia multiply rapidly by *mitosis*, producing thousands of these primitive germ cells. Before birth, all oogonia enlarge to form primary oocytes and most of them have entered the *first meiotic prophase*, but this process remains in an arrested state until puberty.

No oogonia form postnatally. Although several million primary oocytes are present in the fetal ovaries, many of them undergo atresia. About one million primary oocytes are present in each ovary at birth.

Development of the Genital Ducts

Male and female embryos have identical pairs of genital ducts. The male or **mesonephric ducts** play an important part in the development of the male reproductive system. The female or **paramesonephric ducts** develop into the female reproductive system. During the indifferent state of sexual development, both pairs of genital ducts are present.

Development of the Male Genital Ducts (Fig. 12–5A).   The *androgens*, secreted by the fetal testes, are responsible for the differentiation of the male genital ducts. A *müllerian inhibiting substance*, also secreted by the testes, suppresses the development of the **paramesonephric ducts** (müllerian ducts). The mesonephric duct becomes the epididymis, ductus deferens, and ejaculatory duct.

The *seminal vesicle* develops from a diverticulum that arises from the distal end of the mesonephric duct (see Fig. 12–5A). Most of the paramesonephric ducts degenerate, but their cranial tips and those of the mesonephric ducts persist as appendages of the testes and epididymis, respectively.

Development of the Female Genital Ducts (See Fig. 12–5B and C).   In embryos lacking a Y chromosome, the paramesonephric ducts form most of the female genital tract. Their cranial parts form the uterine tubes and their caudal parts fuse to form the **uterovaginal primordium** or canal which develops into the uterus and part of the vagina. Contact of the uterovaginal primordium with the urogenital sinus induces paired endodermal outgrowths, called **sinovaginal bulbs**, to form. These bulbs fuse to form a solid **vaginal plate** (see Fig. 12–5B). The central cells of this plate soon break down, forming the cavity of the vagina; the peripheral cells form the vaginal epithelium. The uterovaginal primordium likely contributes to the superior part of the vagina, but its entire epithelium is probably derived from endodermal cells in the vaginal plate.

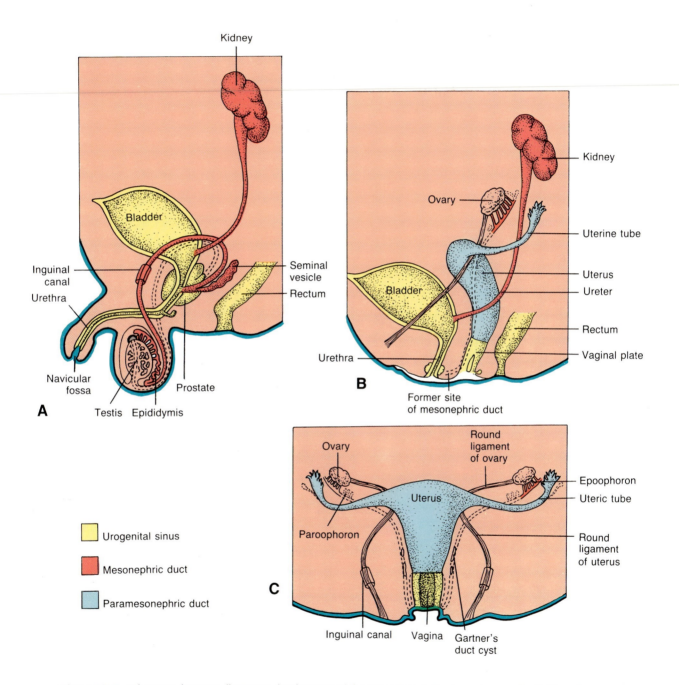

Figure 12–5 Schematic drawings, illustrating development of the internal genitalia. *A*, newborn male; *B*, 12-week female fetus; *C*, newborn female. (Modified from Moore KL. Before we are born. Basic embryology and birth defects. 2nd ed. Philadelphia: WB Saunders, 1983.)

Development of the External Genitalia

The early development of the external genitalia is similar in both sexes. Distinguishing sexual characteristics begin to appear during the ninth week, but the external genital organs are not fully differentiated until the twelfth week.

The Indifferent External Genitalia (Fig. 12–6A and B).   Early in the fourth week, a *genital tubercle* develops at the cranial end of the cloacal membrane.

Labioscrotal swellings and **urogenital folds** soon develop on each side of this membrane. The genital tubercle elongates to form a **phallus** which is similar in both sexes.

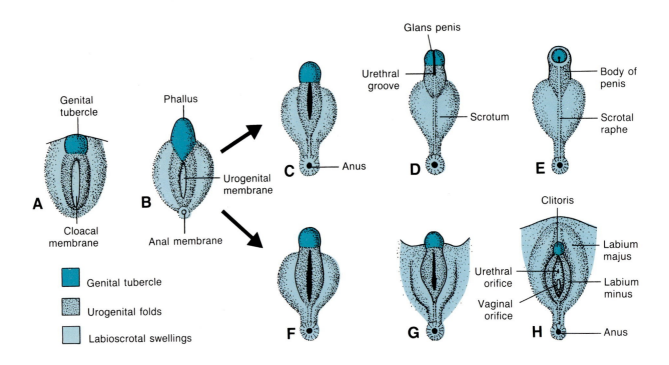

Figure 12–6 Drawings illustrating the development of the external genitalia. *A* and *B*, the indifferent stage; *C* to *E*, stages in the development of male external genitalia at 9, 11, and 12 weeks; *F* to *H*, stages in the development of female genitalia at 9, 11, and 12 weeks. (Modified from Moore KL. The developing human. Clinically oriented embryology. 4th ed. Philadelphia: WB Saunders, 1988.)

Development of the Male External Genitalia (See Fig. 12–6c to E).   Masculinization of the indifferent external genitalia is caused by androgens produced by the fetal testes. As the phallus elongates to form the *penis,* the urogenital folds fuse on the ventral surface of the penis to form the *spongy urethra.* The labioscrotal swellings grow toward the median plane and fuse to form the **scrotum** (see Fig. 12–6E). The line of fusion of the labioscrotal folds is clearly indicated by the *scrotal raphe.*

Development of the Female External Genitalia (See Fig. 12–6F to H). Both the urethra and vagina open into the urogenital sinus which in this region becomes the *vestibule of the vagina.* The urogenital folds become the **labia minora,** the labioscrotal swellings become the **labia majora,** and the phallus becomes the **clitoris.**

Congenital Malformations of the Genital System

Hypospadias.   If fusion of the urogenital folds is incomplete, abnormal openings of the urethra form along the ventral aspect of the penis. This malformation occurs in about one in every 300 infants. Most often, the abnormal urethral orifice is near the glans penis (**glandular hypospadias**). This malformation usually results from failure of canalization of the ectodermal *glandular plate.* This cord-like structure forms in the glans penis and gives rise to the terminal part of the spongy urethra. Glandular hypospadias results from failure of fusion of the distal parts of the urogenital folds. The other common type of hypospadias is called **penile hypospadias.** It also results from defective closure of the urogenital folds. As a consequence, the urethra opens on the ventral surface of the body (shaft) of the penis.

Malformations of the Uterus and Vagina.   As the formation of the uterus depends upon the fusion of the two paramesonephric ducts (see Fig. 12–5B), various forms of duplication of the uterus result when this fusion is incomplete. Complete failure of the fusion of these ducts will give rise to a duplication of the entire female genital tract (*double uterus and double vagina*). Rarely, one paramesonephric duct fails to develop. This results in the formation of a single uterine tube and a single horn of the uterus (**unicornuate uterus**).

Descent of the Gonads

As the mesonephric kidneys degenerate (see Fig. 12–2A), the gonads descend from the abdomen to the pelvis. As this occurs, a diverticulum of the peritoneum, called the **processus vaginalis,** protrudes through the anterior abdominal wall to form the primordium of the inguinal canal. The processus vaginalis is attached posteriorly to the *gubernaculum,* a ligament that extends from the caudal pole of the gonad to the labioscrotal swelling.

In the male, the testes remain near the deep inguinal rings until about the twenty-eighth week. Then they quickly descend through the inguinal canals and usually enter the scrotum before birth. The distal part of the processus vaginalis persists as the *tunica vaginalis* of the testis; the remainder of this process normally disappears.

In *the female*, the gubernaculum attaches to the uterus forming the *ovarian ligament* proximal to this attachment (see Fig. 12–5C) and the *round ligament* distal to it. Normally the processus vaginalis completely obliterates.

Cryptorchidism and Ectopic Testes.   Failure of the testes to descend into the scrotum (*cryptorchidism*) and maldescent of the testes during which the testes descend to an abnormal position (*ectopic testes*) are the most common malformations of the male genital system. The testes may remain anywhere between the abdomen and the scrotum. Ectopic testes may be in the perineum, anterior to the pubis, or in the thighs.

INTERSEXUALITY

Because an embryo has the potential to develop as either a male or a female, errors in sex development result in various degrees of intermediate sex, a condition known as **intersexuality** or **hermaphroditism**. A person with ambiguous external genitalia is called an intersex or a hermaphrodite. Intersexual individuals are classified according to the histologic appearance of their gonads.

True Hermaphrodites.   Persons with this very rare condition have both ovarian and testicular tissues. The internal and external genitalia are variable. Most true hermaphrodites have a 46, XX karyotype (chromosome set), but some are mosaics (46, XX/46, XY).

Female Pseudohermaphrodites.   Persons with this condition have a 46, XX karyotype. The most common cause of female pseudohermaphroditism is **congenital virilizing adrenal hyperplasia.** Several types occur, all of which are inherited as autosomal recessives. During fetal development there is an increased secretion of ACTH (adrenocorticotropic hormone) and hyperplasia of the suprarenal (adrenal) glands. The resulting production of androgens leads to masculinization of the external genitalia (enlarged clitoris, abnormalities of the urogenital sinus, and partial fusion of the labia majora).

The external genitalia of a female fetus may also be masculinized by androgenic hormones that reach it via the placenta from the maternal circulation. These hormones may be present in excessive amounts if the mother's suprarenal cortices are overactive, or if she has received hormone therapy involving androgenic substances.

Male Pseudohermaphrodites.   Individuals with this condition have testes and a 46, XY karyotype. The external and internal genitalia are variable owing to varying degrees of development of the penis and the genital ducts. This condition results from an inadequate production of androgens by the fetal testes, or when the embryonic genital tissues do not respond to the male hormones.

CARDIOVASCULAR SYSTEM

CARDIOVASCULAR SYSTEM

THE VASCULAR SYSTEM

Development of Blood Vessels

The human embryo can obtain sufficient nourishment during the second week of development by diffusion of nutrients from the maternal blood flowing through the **lacunar networks** in the **syncytiotrophoblast** (see Chapter 2 and Fig. 2–1C). As the embryo increases in size, a more efficient system for supplying nourishment and exchanging gases (e.g., O_2 and CO_2) is required.

The vascular system begins during the third week in the wall of the yolk sac. Groups of mesenchymal cells, called **angioblasts**, form **blood islands** (see Chapter 3 and Fig. 3–4A). As cavities develop in these islands, primitive blood cells and vessels form. The primitive blood vessels join to form a vascular network in the wall of the yolk sac. Blood vessels form in a similar manner in the mesenchyme associated with the connecting stalk and chorion, including its villi. Blood vessels also form in the embryo towards the end of the third week and join to form a continuous system of vessels on each side.

Blood vessels in the embryo soon join those on the yolk sac and in the connecting stalk and chorion to form a **primitive cardiovascular system** (Fig. 13–1A). **Cardinal veins** return blood from the embryo; **vitelline veins** return blood from the yolk sac, and **umbilical veins** return *oxygenated blood* from the placenta (see Fig. 3–4B). Only one umbilical vein persists. Initially there are also two **dorsal aortae** (see Fig. 13–1A), but these soon fuse in the caudal half of the embryo to form a single dorsal aorta (see Fig. 13–1B).

The Aortic Arches

Each branchial arch is supplied by an artery called an aortic arch (see Figs. 9–1C, 13–1, and 13–2A), although the arteries to the fifth pair of arches are often rudimentary or absent. As the adult arterial pattern develops, the original aortic arch arteries are transformed into new vessels (see Fig. 13–2B).

Derivatives of the Aortic Arches. The **third pair of aortic arches** becomes the *common carotid arteries* and the proximal parts of the *internal carotid arteries* (see Fig. 13–2B). The fourth pair of aortic arches persists, but its derivatives differ on the two sides. The **left fourth aortic arch** forms part of the *arch of the aorta*, whereas the **right fourth aortic arch** forms the proximal part of the *right subclavian artery* (see Fig. 13–2B).

The derivatives of the sixth pair of aortic arches also differ on the two sides.

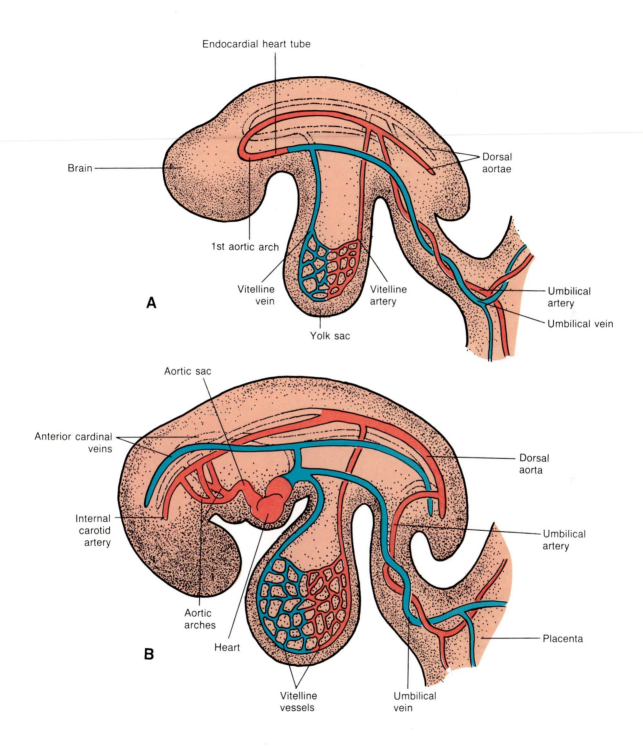

Figure 13-1 *A*, drawing of the primitive cardiovascular system in an embryo of about 21 days. The future heart is represented by two endocardial heart tubes. Each tube is continuous with the first aortic arch, the artery of the first branchial arch (see Figs. 9–1 and 9–2); *B*, drawing of the cardiovascular system in an embryo of about 26 days. The heart tubes have fused to form a tubular heart (see Fig. 13–3). The umbilical vein carries oxygenated blood and nutrients to the embryo from the placenta.

The **right sixth aortic arch** becomes the *right pulmonary artery*, whereas the **left sixth aortic arch** forms the *left pulmonary artery* and the **ductus arteriosus** (see Fig. 13–2B). The ductus arteriosus shunts most of the blood in the pulmonary trunk to the aorta because the lungs are nonfunctional and require very little blood.

Common aortic arch abnormalities include **patent ductus arteriosus** and **coarctation of the aorta**. In the latter condition, the aortic lumen is narrowed inferior to the origin of the left subclavian artery. Abnormal origin of the right subclavian artery, double aortic arch, and right aorta occur infrequently. (For details about these malformations, see Moore KL. The developing human. Clinically oriented embryology. 4th ed. Philadelphia: WB Saunders, 1988:321).

THE HEART

Development of the Heart

The earliest indication of heart development is the appearance of **cardiogenic cords** of cells in the cardiogenic area (see Fig. 3–4A). These cords of mesenchymal cells soon become canalized to form two thin-walled, endothelial tubes called **endocardial heart tubes** (see Figs. 13–1A and 13–3A). Located in the floor of the future pericardial cavity, these tubes soon fuse to form a single **heart tube** (see Figs. 13–1B and 13–3B). The splanchnic mesenchyme adjacent to this tubular heart condenses to form the primordia of the *myocardium* and *epicardium* of the heart wall.

The following series of constrictions and dilations soon appear in the heart and indicate distinct regions (see Fig. 13–3B and C): (1) the **sinus venosus**, the caudal region of the primitive heart, receives all the blood returning to the heart from the *common cardinal veins, vitelline veins*, and *umbilical veins*; (2) the **primitive atrium**; (3) the **primitive ventricle**; (4) the **bulbus cordis**, and (5) the **truncus arteriosus** (see Fig. 13–3C and D).

The sinus venosus is partly embedded in the **septum transversum** (the primordium of the central tendon of the diaphragm; see Figs. 8–2 and 13–3A), whereas the **truncus arteriosus** dilates to form the **aortic sac** from which the **aortic arches** arise (see Figs. 13–1B and 13–2A). These arteries pass dorsally and enter the **branchial arches** (see Chapter 9 and Fig. 9–1C). The aortic arches open into the corresponding dorsal aorta (see Fig. 13–1A and B). The primitive heart tube grows rapidly and bends upon itself because it is fixed at its cranial and caudal ends. This bending forms a U-shaped *bulboventricular loop* (see Fig. 13–3D).

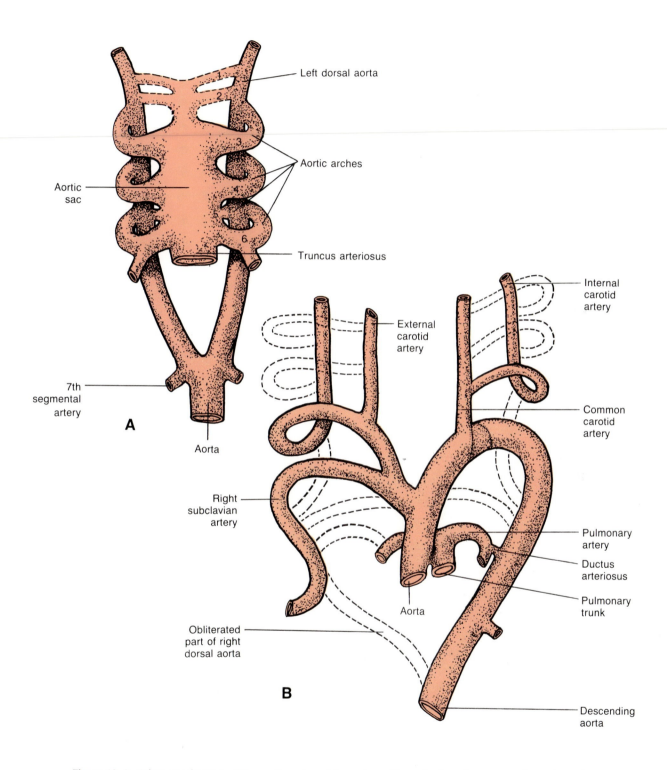

Left dorsal aorta

Aortic arches

Aortic sac

Truncus arteriosus

7th segmental artery

A

Aorta

Internal carotid artery

External carotid artery

Common carotid artery

Right subclavian artery

Pulmonary artery

Ductus arteriosus

Pulmonary trunk

Aorta

Obliterated part of right dorsal aorta

B

Descending aorta

Figure 13–2 Schematic drawings of the aortic arches of the embryo, illustrating how they are transformed into the adult arterial pattern. *A*, aortic arches in a six-week embryo; *B*, the arterial arrangement in an eight-week embryo. (Modified from Moore KL. The developing human. Clinically oriented embryology. 4th ed. Philadelphia: WB Saunders, 1988).

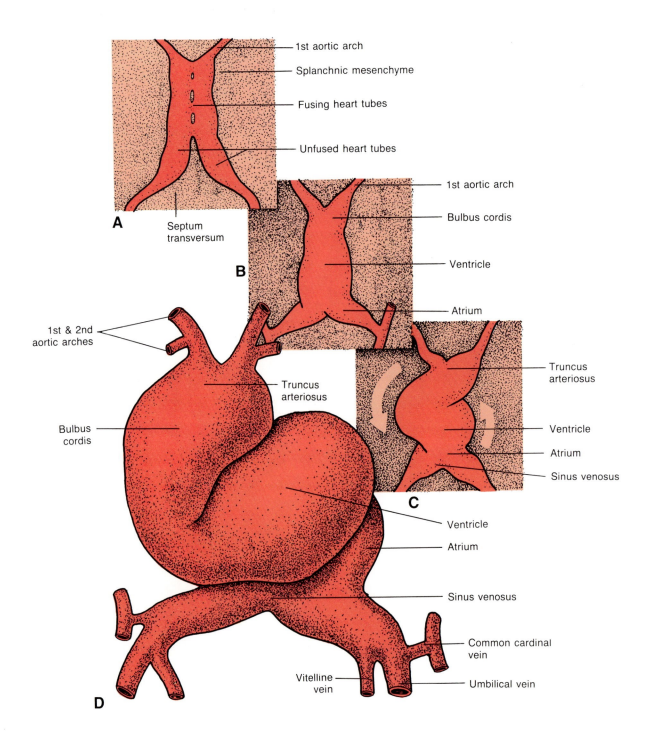

Figure 13–3 Drawings of ventral views of the developing heart during the fourth week. Note that the endocardial heart tubes gradually fuse to form a single tubular heart. The fusion begins at the cranial end of the tubes and extends caudally until a single tubular heart is formed. As the heart elongates, it bends upon itself, forming an S-shaped heart as shown in *D*.

Fate of the Sinus Venosus and Formation of the Adult Right Atrium.   The sinus venosus is initially a separate chamber of the primitive heart that opens into the right atrium (Fig. 13–3D). As development of the heart proceeds, the **left horn** of the sinus venosus becomes the *coronary sinus* and its **right horn** is incorporated into the wall of the right atrium, where it forms the smooth portion of the adult right atrial wall. The right half of the primitive atrium persists as the *right auricle*, the appendage of the atrium (see Fig. 13–4D).

Formation of the Adult Left Atrium.   Most of the adult left atrium is formed by incorporation of the *primitive pulmonary vein*. As the atrium enlarges, parts of this vein and its branches are absorbed, with the result that four pulmonary veins eventually enter the adult left atrium. The smooth-walled part of the left atrium is derived from absorbed pulmonary vein tissue (see Fig. 13–4C), whereas the left auricle is derived from the primitive atrium.

Formation of the Four-Chambered Heart

During the fourth and fifth weeks, the primitive heart is divided into the typical four-chambered human organ.

Division of the Atrioventricular Canal.   Two localized proliferations of mesenchyme, called *endocardial cushions*, develop in the atrioventricular region of the heart (see Fig. 13–4A). These cushions grow toward each other and fuse, dividing the atrioventricular canal into right and left atrioventricular (AV) canals (see Fig. 13–4C).

Division of the Primitive Atrium.   A sickle-shaped, membranous partition (see Fig. 13–4A and B), known as the **septum primum**, grows from the dorsal wall of the primitive atrium. It eventually fuses with the merged endocardial cushions (see Fig. 13–4A and B). Before the septum primum fuses with these cushions, a communication exists between the right and left halves of the primitive atrium through the *ostium primum* or **foramen primum** (see Fig. 13–4A).

As the septum primum fuses with the endocardial cushions, obliterating the foramen primum, the superior part of the septum primum breaks down, creating another opening called the **foramen secundum** (see Fig. 13–4B). As this round foramen develops, another sickle-shaped, membranous fold, called the **septum secundum**, grows into the atrium to the right of the septum primum (see Fig. 13–3B). The septum secundum overlaps the foramen secundum, the opening in the septum primum. There is also an opening between the free edge of the septum secundum and the dorsal wall of the atrium. It is called the **foramen ovale** (see Fig. 13–4C). By this stage, the remains of the septum primum has formed the flap-like valve of the foramen ovale.

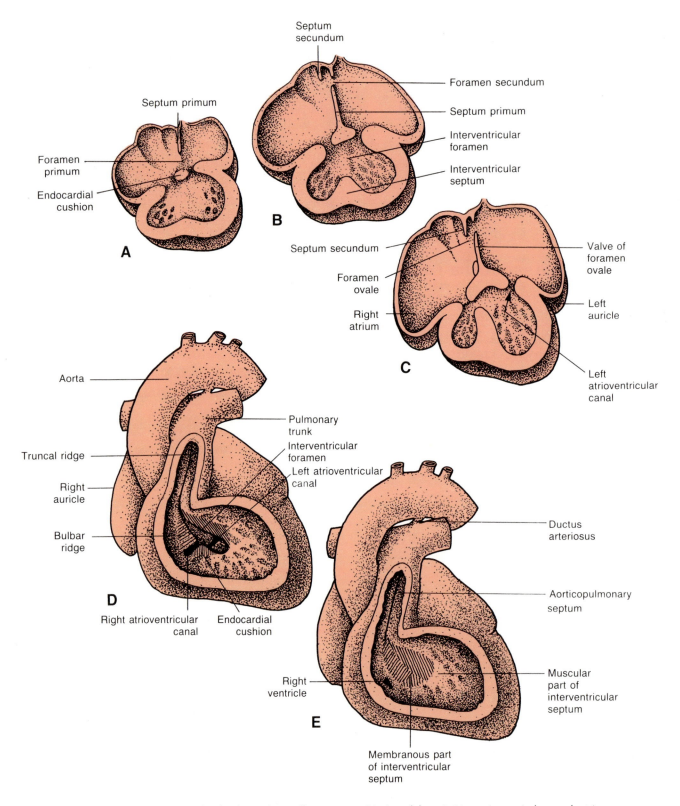

Figure 13-4   Drawings of the developing heart, illustrating partitioning of the primitive atrioventricular canal, atrium, and ventricle. *A, B,* and *C* are frontal sections of the embryonic heart during the fourth week; *D* and *E* are schematic drawings of the heart illustrating closure of the interventricular foramen and formation of the interventricular septum; *D,* five weeks; *E,* seven weeks. Note that the interventricular foramen is closed by tissues from three sources. (Modified from Moore KL. The developing human. Clinically oriented embryology. 4th ed. Philadelphia: WB Saunders 1988).

Atrial septal defects result from abnormal development of the interatrial septum. The common defect is characterized by a large opening in the septum between the right and left atria (**persistent foramen ovale**). This defect results from (1) excessive absorption of the septum primum, or (2) underdevelopment of the septum secundum, or (3) a combination of these abnormalities.

Formation of the Ventricles. The primitive ventricle (see Fig. 13–4A) gives rise to most of the left ventricle, whereas the bulbus cordis forms most of the right ventricle. The *interventricular septum* begins as a ridge in the floor of the primitive ventricle (see Fig. 13–4B) and slowly grows toward the endocardial cushions. Until the end of the seventh week, the future right and left ventricles communicate through a large **interventricular foramen** (see Fig. 13–4B and C). Closure of the interventricular foramen results in the formation of the membranous part of the interventricular septum. This part is derived from the fusion of tissue from the endocardial cushions and bulbar ridges (see Fig. 13–4D and E).

Partitioning of the Bulbus Cordis and Truncus Arteriosus. Division of these parts of the primitive heart results from the development and fusion of the **truncal ridges** and **bulbar ridges** (see Fig. 13–4D). The fused mesenchymal ridges form an **aorticopulmonary septum** that divides the truncus arteriosus and bulbus cordis into the *ascending aorta* and the *pulmonary trunk* (see Fig. 13–3D and E).

Abnormalities in the formation of the aorticopulmonary septum result in the following major congenital malformations: **transposition of the great arteries (vessels), persistent truncus arteriosus**, and **ventricular septal defects**. Ventricular septal defects, the most common congenital heart malformation, are usually in the membranous part of the interventricular septum.

Development of the Conducting System of the Heart. The sinoatrial node initially forms in the wall of the sinus venosus, near its opening into the right atrium (see Fig. 13–3D). The *sinoatrial node* is later incorporated into the right atrium with the right horn of the sinus venosus.

The *atrioventricular node and bundle* are derived from cells in the walls of sinus venosus and atrioventricular canal.

CARDIOVASCULAR CHANGES AFTER BIRTH

Changes in the Circulation of Blood at Birth. At birth the lungs expand and the blood flow to them increases rapidly. They take over oxygen and carbon dioxide exchange when the placenta separates from the newborn infant. *The ductus arteriosus and foramen ovale close.* When blood pressure in the left atrium increases at birth, the flap-like septum primum is pressed against the relatively rigid septum secundum. As a result, *the foramen ovale closes* and communication between the atria normally ceases.

Various other fetal vessels also lose their functions and become ligamentous. The derivatives of these vessels appear in italics: **ductus arteriosus** (*ligamentum arteriosum*); **umbilical vein** (*ligamentum teres*); **ductus venosus** (*ligamentum venosum*), and **umbilical arteries** (*medial umbilical ligaments*).

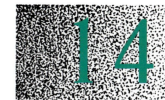

ARTICULAR AND SKELETAL SYSTEMS

ARTICULAR AND SKELETAL SYSTEMS

The articular and skeletal systems develop from mesoderm. The embryonic mesoderm adjacent to the developing notochord (embryonic axis) and neural tube thickens to form two longitudinal columns called **paraxial mesoderm** (Fig. 14–1A). These mesodermal columns are soon divided into paired segments called **somites** (see Fig. 14–1B). The somites form elevations on the dorsolateral surface of the embryo (see Chapter 4 and Fig. 4–3). Each somite consists of a **sclerotome** and a **dermomyotome** (see Fig. 14–1C). Mesenchymal cells leave the sclerotomes and envelop the notochord. Here they give rise to the vertebral column and ribs. Mesenchymal cells from the **myotome regions** of the dermomyotome give rise to the back muscles (see Figs. 14–1D and 15–1D). The **dermatome regions** of the dermomyotomes give rise to the dermis of the skin.

BONES

Bone Development

Bones are first indicated by condensations of mesenchymal cells that form mesenchymal models of the bones. Some bones develop in this mesenchyme (embryonic connective tissue) by **intramembranous bone formation.** In other cases, the mesenchymal bone models are transformed into cartilage models of the bones in the following manner. The mesenchymal cells that have aggregated in the shape of the bone to be formed differentiate into embryonic cartilage cells, called **chondroblasts.** These cells secrete cartilage matrix so that the bone model soon consists of hyaline cartilage. The cartilage bone model is later ossified by **endochondral bone formation.**

Bone development is known as *ossification* or **osteogenesis.** There are two different mechanisms of osteogenesis. *All bones are derived from mesenchyme,* but by two different processes, depending on which bones are involved. For example the flat bones of the skull cap, or calvaria (Fig. 14–3), develop directly in areas of vascularized mesenchyme by a process known as **intramembranous ossification.** The process was so named because the site of these bones is first indicated by a mesenchymal membrane. Long bones, as mentioned previously, are preceded by cartilage models (see Fig. 16–2 on page 152). Most of the cartilage in these bones is replaced during fetal life by bone tissue during a process known as **endochondral ossification.**

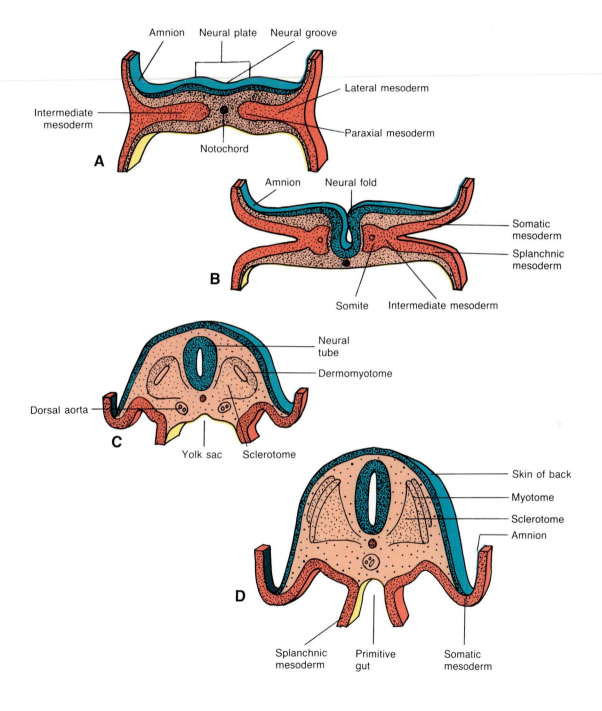

Figure 14–1 Transverse sections through embryos at various stages, illustrating the formation and differentiation of the somites. *A*, about 18 days; *B*, about 22 days; *C*, about 24 days; *D*, about 26 days. Note that cells from the sclerotome regions of the somites migrate toward the notochord, where they aggregate to form the mesenchymal model of a vertebra (see Fig. 14–2A).

THE AXIAL SKELETON

Development of The Vertebral Column

Vertebrae are derived from the sclerotome regions of the somites (see Fig. 14–1C and D). Mesenchymal cells from these regions migrate toward the median plane and surround the notochord (see Fig. 14–2A). Each vertebra forms from the condensation of mesenchymal cells from the caudal half of one sclerotome which fuses with loosely arranged mesenchymal cells from the cranial half of the next sclerotome.

The notochord persists throughout the mesenchymal and cartilaginous stages of vertebral development, but eventually disappears as ossification of the vertebrae occurs (Fig. 14–2). The adult derivative of the notochord is the **nucleus pulposus,** which forms the central part of an intervertebral disc.

As development proceeds, processes arise from the developing vertebra: a spinous process, a vertebral arch, two transverse processes, and two costal processes. The processes that form the vertebral arch (neural arch) grow dorsomedially and fuse with each other in the median plane to enclose the developing spinal cord. Failure of these processes to meet and fuse results in the formation of a bony defect in the vertebral arch known as **spina bifida occulta** (see Fig. 17–4A). If the vertebral arches of several vertebrae fail to develop normally, the combined bony defects may allow the meninges (membranes) and spinal cord to herniate (see Fig. 17–4B and C), producing a severe form of spina bifida, known as **spina bifida cystica** (e.g., meningocele and meningomyelocele).

The transverse processes grow laterally from the vertebrae and the costal processes grow ventrolaterally into the body wall. In the thoracic region, the costal processes form the ribs (see Fig. 14–2D).

During or shortly after puberty (12 to 16 years), five secondary centers of ossification appear in the vertebrae (see Fig. 14–2E). All secondary centers unite with the rest of the vertebra at about 25 years.

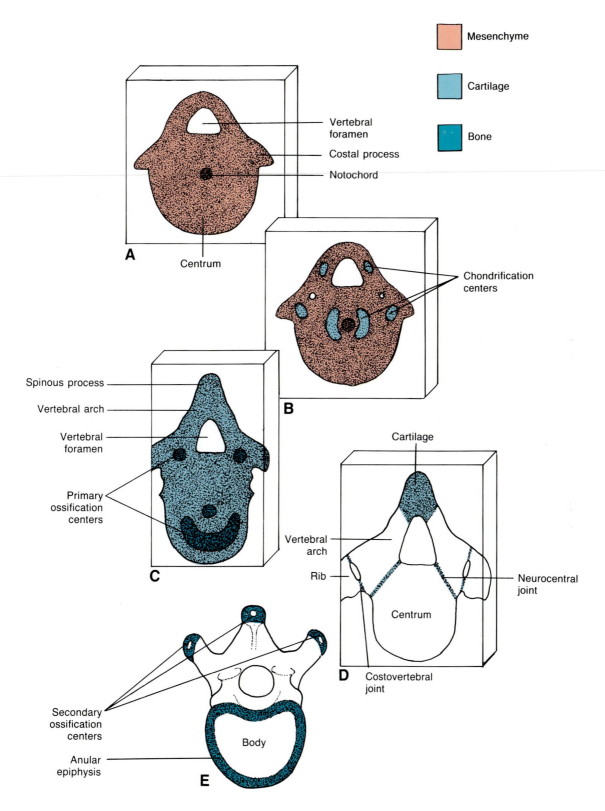

Figure 14-2 Drawings illustrating various stages in the development of a vertebra; *A*, mesenchymal stage at five weeks; *B*, chondrification centers in a mesenchymal vertebra at six weeks; *C*, primary ossification centers in a cartilaginous vertebra at seven weeks; *D*, a thoracic vertebra at birth. Note that it consists of three bony parts: a centrum and two halves of the vertebral arch (neural arch); *E*, a thoracic vertebra in a child of about 12 years, showing the location of the secondary centers of ossification. There are two anular (annular) epiphyses: one on the inferior and one on the superior rim of the body of the vertebra.

Development of the Skull

The skull develops from two parts: a neurocranium and a viscerocranium (see Fig. 14–3). The **neurocranium** is divided into (1) a *membranous neurocranium* which gives rise to the flat bones of the skull (e.g., the parietal bones) which surround the brain and form the calvaria (cranial vault), and (2) a *cartilaginous neurocranium*, or chondrocranium, which forms the base of the skull.

At birth, the flat bones of the skull are separated from each other by connective tissue *sutures*. In areas where more than two bones meet, the sutures are wide and are known as **fontanelles** (see Fig. 5–2). The most prominent of these is the anterior fontanelle which is located where the two parietal bones meet the two parts of the frontal bone. The sutures and fontanelles of the skull permit the bones of the skull to overlap each other during birth which enables the head to pass through the birth canal (cervical canal and vagina). Several of these sutures and fontanelles remain membranous for a considerable time after birth. For example, the **anterior fontanelle** (often called the "soft spot") usually closes by the middle of the second year.

The **viscerocranium** forms the bones of the face and is derived mainly from the cartilages of the first two branchial arches (see Fig. 14–3). See Chapter 9 for a description of the branchial apparatus and its derivatives.

Skull Malformations. When there are severe malformations of the brain (e.g., *meroanencephaly*, absence of most of the brain; see Fig. 17–5A), the flat bones of the skull fail to form. This condition is called **acrania.**

Premature closure of the cranial sutures results in severe deformities in the shape of the skull, such as **scaphocephaly** (long narrow skull), and **oxycephaly** or turricephaly (tower-like skull).

THE APPENDICULAR SKELETON

Development of the Appendicular Skeleton

The appendicular skeleton consists of the pectoral (shoulder) and pelvic girdles and the limb bones. The limb bones initially appear as mesenchymal condensations in the fifth week (see Fig. 16–2B). After chondrification centers develop, cartilaginous models of the bones develop in the sixth week (see Fig. 16–2C).

Primary ossification centers develop in these long bones and ossification begins by the end of the embryonic period (56 days). By the twelfth week primary centers have appeared in nearly all the limb bones.

Secondary ossification centers usually appear just before birth in the bones that form the knee joint. However, most secondary ossification centers appear after birth.

The bone formed from a primary center does not fuse with the bone formed from the secondary center until the bone reaches its adult length. Knowledge concerning the times of appearance of the various ossification centers is used by radiologists to determine whether the skeleton of a child is growing normally.

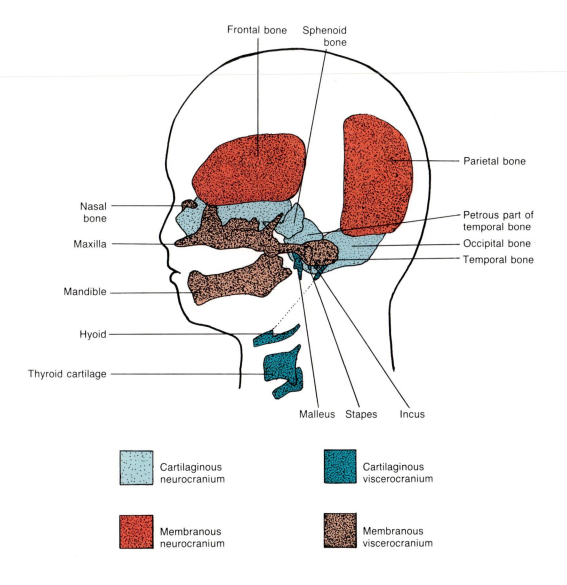

Figure 14–3 A drawing of the fetal skull at 20 weeks, indicating the derivation of its bones. The skull can be divided into two parts: the neurocranium which forms a protective case (the calvaria) around the brain, as shown in Fig. 5–2, and a viscerocranium which forms the skeleton of the face.

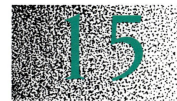

MUSCULAR SYSTEM

MUSCULAR SYSTEM

Most of the muscular system is derived from the **embryonic mesoderm** (Fig. 15–1). The dilator and sphincter pupillae muscles of the iris develop from ectoderm (see page 172).

SKELETAL MUSCLE

Mesenchymal cells leave the **myotome regions** of the **somites** (see Fig. 15–1A) and become elongated, spindle-shaped cells called **myoblasts.** These embryonic muscle cells fuse to form multinucleated muscle cells called muscle fibers. **Myofibrils** soon appear in the cytoplasm of these developing muscle cells and cross-striations develop shortly thereafter. As a result, typical striated muscle cells (fibers) form.

A similar process occurs in the ventrolateral body walls, where the mesenchymal cells are derived from the somatic layer of mesoderm (see Fig. 15–1A). This **somatic mesoderm** layer gives rise to the striated muscles of the body walls and the limbs (see Fig. 15–1B and C).

Myoblasts that develop from mesenchymal cells in the **occipital myotomes** (see Fig. 15–1B) migrate ventrally and form the *extrinsic* and *intrinsic tongue muscles.* These muscles are supplied by the *hypoglossal nerve* (CN XII), which is derived from the occipital group of segmental nerves.

Mesenchymal cells arising from mesoderm around the *prochordal plate* (see Chapter 2) are thought to give rise to the **preotic myotomes.** Myoblasts from these myotomes are thought to form the *extrinsic muscles of the eye* (see Fig. 15–1B).

Mesenchymal cells in the **branchial arches** differentiate into myoblasts that give rise to the *head and neck muscles* (see Chapter 9). These muscles are innervated by the nerve supplying the branchial arch from which the mesenchymal cells are derived (see Table 9–1). For example, the *muscles of facial expression* are supplied by the *facial nerve* (CN VII), the nerve that supplies the second branchial arch.

Most skeletal muscle develops before birth and nearly all the remaining muscles are formed by the end of the first year. Muscle tissue enlarges due to the increase in the diameter of the individual cells. The latter results from the formation of more myofilaments within each fiber.

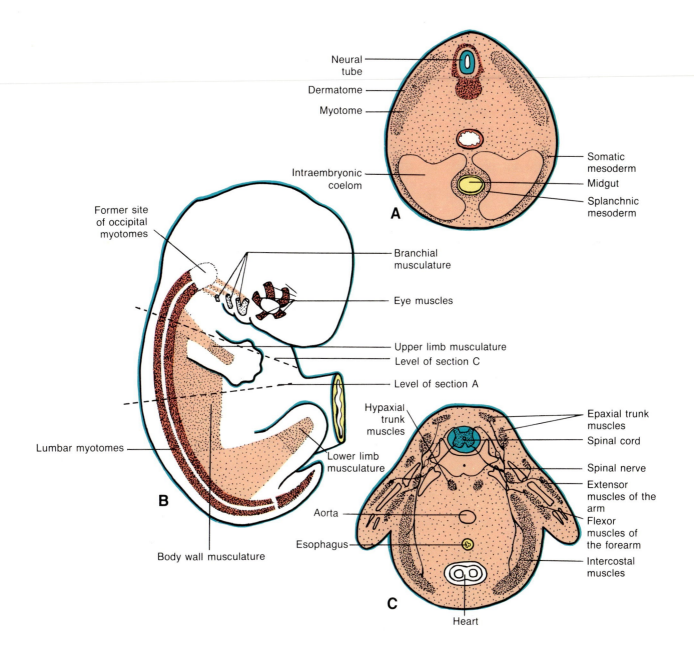

Figure 15–1 *A*, Diagrammatic transverse section through a 28-day embryo, showing the cells of the myotome adjacent to the dermatome. Some cells have migrated from the lateral mesoderm (see Fig. 14–1) and gathered around the intraembryonic coelom to form the somatic mesoderm. Mesenchymal cells in this layer will differentiate into myoblasts (primitive muscle cells) that will form the body wall musculature; *B*, sketch of a lateral view of an embryo during the sixth week, showing the myotomes and the developing muscles; *C*, transverse section of a six-week embryo, illustrating the epaxial and hypaxial derivatives of the myotomes. The limb muscles are not derived from the myotomes; they are derived from the somatic layer of lateral mesoderm (see Fig. 14–1A).

SMOOTH MUSCLE

Most smooth muscle tissue differentiates from mesenchymal cells that are derived from the **splanchnic mesoderm** layer surrounding the primitive gut and its derivatives (see Fig. 15–1A).

CARDIAC MUSCLE

Cardiac muscle tissue is derived from the **splanchnic mesoderm** that surrounds the primitive heart (see Fig. 13–3A). The myoblasts adhere to each other and later *intercalated discs* develop at their junctions, but the myoblasts do not fuse. Myofibrils develop in embryonic cardiac muscle cells in the same manner as in skeletal muscle. A few special bundles of muscle cells with irregularly distributed myofibrils develop. These bundles of cells give rise to the *Purkinje fibers,* which form the conducting system of the heart. (For details, see page 308 in Moore KL. The developing human. Clinically oriented embryology. 4th ed. Philadelphia: WB Saunders, 1988.)

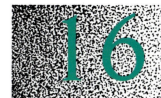

16

LIMBS

LIMBS

Limb Development

The limbs develop as outgrowths of the ventrolateral body wall toward the end of the fourth week (see Figs. 4–3 and 16–1A). The **limb buds**, the earliest rudiments of the limbs, result from localized proliferations of the somatic mesoderm. The upper limb buds are visible by day 26 or 27 and the lower limb buds are recognizable by day 28. The limb buds elongate by the proliferation of mesenchyme within them.

The early stages of limb development are alike for the upper and lower limbs, except that the development of the upper limb buds precedes that of the lower limb buds by a few days (Fig. 16–1). The upper limb buds develop opposite the caudal cervical segments and the lower limb buds appear opposite the lumbar and cranial sacral segments.

Each limb bud consists of a core of mesenchyme, derived from the somatic mesoderm layer, and a covering layer of surface ectoderm. At the tip of each limb bud, the ectodermal cells multiply to form a localized thickening known as the **apical ectodermal ridge** (Fig. 16–2A). This ridge exerts an inductive influence on the limb mesenchyme that results in the rapid growth and development of the limbs.

During the fifth week, the distal ends of the flipper-like limb buds flatten to form paddle-shaped **hand and foot plates** (see Fig. 16–1B). By the end of the sixth week, some of the mesenchymal tissue in the hand plates condenses to form **digital rays** which outline the pattern of the digits (see Fig. 16–1C). During the seventh week, similar mesenchymal digital rays develop in the foot plates. Notches soon appear between the digital rays, first in the hand plates and later in the foot plates (see Fig. 16–1D). Tissue breakdown occurs in the clefts between the digital rays (see Fig. 16–1E). This process produces separate digits (fingers and toes) during the eighth week (see Fig. 16–1F).

As the developing limbs elongate, the bones form. First, a mesenchymal skeleton is formed as the cells aggregate to form the primordia of the bones in the developing limbs during the early part of the fifth week (see Fig. 16–2B). **Chondrification centers** appear later in the fifth week (see Fig. 16–2C), and by the end of the sixth week the entire skeleton of the limbs is cartilaginous (see Fig. 16–2D).

Osteogenesis or ossification of the long bones of the limbs begins in the seventh week from **primary ossification centers** located in the middle of the long bones. Ossification of the long bones is well advanced at 12 weeks. Ossification of the carpal (wrist) bones does not usually begin until the first year after birth.

Most of the *limb musculature* differentiates in situ from mesenchymal cells surrounding the bones. As the bones develop, myoblasts aggregate and form a

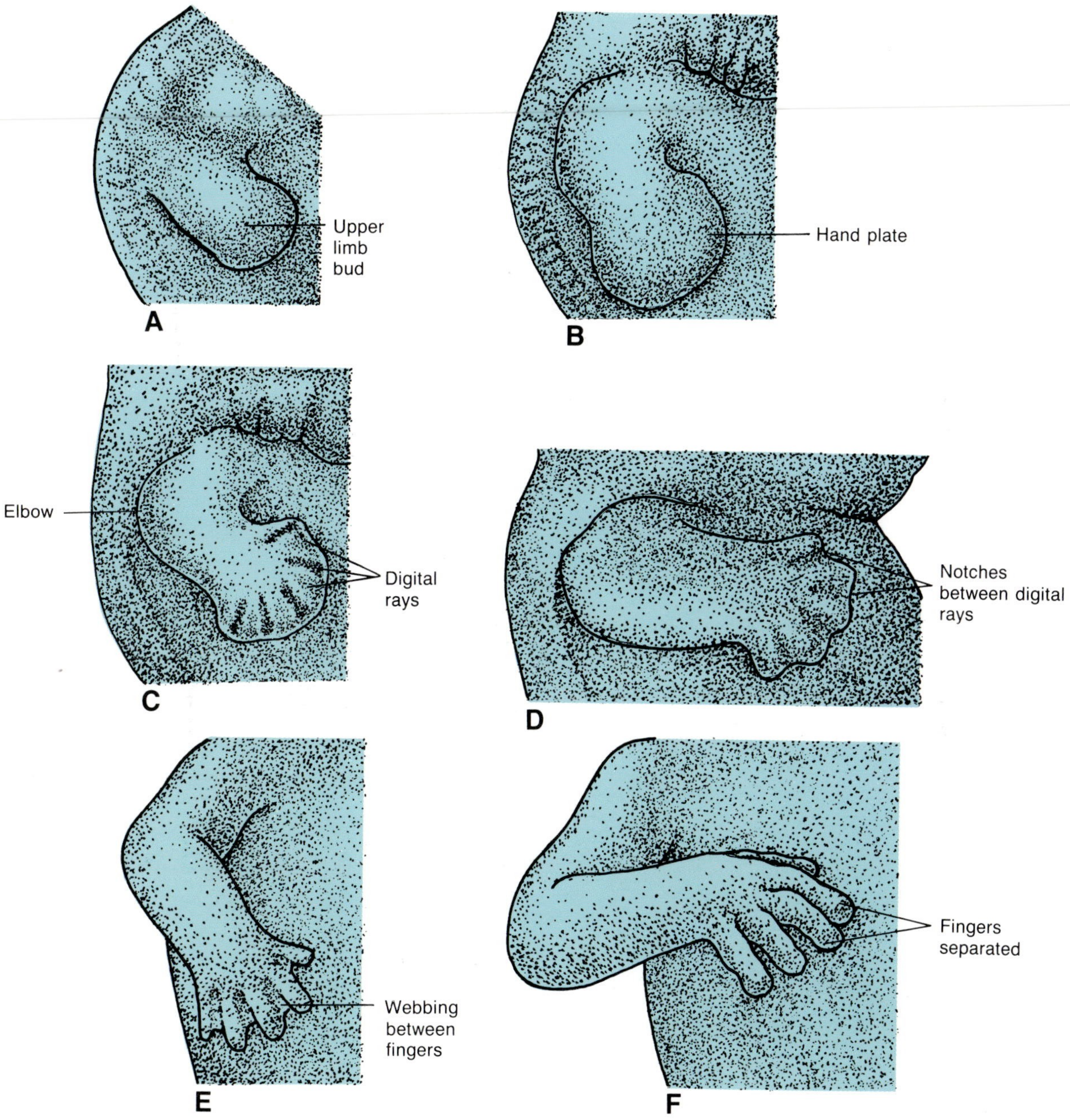

Figure 16–1 Drawings illustrating the various stages of the developing upper limbs. *A*, 32 days; *B*, 36 days; *C*, 41 days; *D*, 48 days; *E*, 51 days; *F*, 56 days. Development of the lower limbs is similar, but occurs a day or so later.

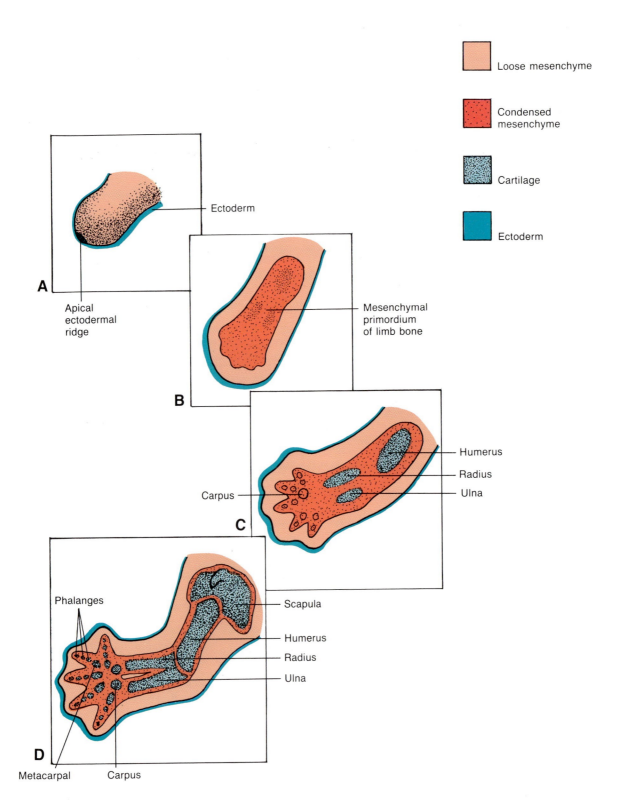

Figure 16-2 Drawings illustrating the development of the skeleton of the upper limb. *A*, 4 weeks; *B*, 5 weeks; *C*, early sixth week; *D*, late sixth week. It is the apical ectodermal ridge *(A)* that exerts the inductive influence on the limb mesenchyme, which, in turn, promotes growth and development of the limb.

large muscle mass in each limb bud. In general, these muscle masses separate into dorsal (extensor) and ventral (flexor) components (see Fig. 15–1C). At first, the upper and lower limb buds are relatively high on the trunk. Here they are invaded by the ventral rami of the adjacent spinal nerves, C5 to T1 and L2 to S3, respectively. The limbs descend during the sixth to eighth weeks, bringing them into their normal relationship to the trunk.

Initially, the developing limbs are directed caudally. Later, they project ventrally and rotate on their longitudinal axes. The upper and lower limbs rotate in opposite directions and to different degrees. Consequently, the future elbow regions point posteriorly and the future knee regions face anteriorly.

The **dermatomes** of the limbs form the dermis of the skin. The cutaneous branches of the main nerve trunks supply the dermatomes in a segmental manner.

Limb Malformations

Minor limb defects are relatively common (e.g., an extra digit), but major limb malformations are uncommon. The critical period of limb development is from 24 to 42 days after fertilization. Many severe limb malformations occurred from 1957 to 1962 owing to the maternal ingestion of *thalidomide*, a potent teratogenic agent. This drug, widely used as a sedative and antinauseant, was withdrawn from the market in December, 1961. Since that time, severe limb malformations have rarely been observed. The term **amelia** indicates complete absence of a limb or limbs, whereas **meromelia** denotes partial absence of a limb or limbs (e.g., absence of a hand or foot).

The lobster-claw malformation results from the failure of the central digital ray to develop. As a result, the middle metacarpal (or metatarsal) and middle digit are absent. This results in a deep central cleft in the hand or foot.

Syndactyly (fusion of adjacent digits) results when the degenerative process responsible for the formation of separate digits fails to occur (see Fig. 16–1D and E). Simple syndactyly is represented by a webbing of the affected fingers or toes. In more severe cases there is fusion of the adjacent digits; there may even be fusion of the bones (synostosis).

Club foot (talipes) is a common foot malformation, having an incidence of about one in 1,500 infants. This malformation is characterized by abnormal positions of the foot (e.g., inverted). Some cases are examples of a postural deformity resulting from compression of the feet against the wall of the uterus during the final stages of pregnancy. This causes the feet to assume an abnormal position. In most cases, the normal shape of the foot is restored spontaneously after birth. Club foot usually results from *multifactorial inheritance*, that is, the deformity is caused by a combination of factors, genetic and nongenetic, each with only a minor effect.

In **achondroplasia**, endochondral bone formation in the limbs is abnormal, resulting in *impaired growth of the limbs*. This causes the type of dwarfism in which the limbs are disproportionately short in relation to the trunk. The head is also abnormally formed owing to disturbed endochondral bone formation in the base of the skull.

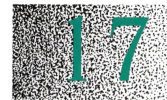

17

NERVOUS SYSTEM

NERVOUS SYSTEM

ORIGINS OF THE NERVOUS SYSTEM

The first indication of the nervous system is the **neural plate**, a thickened area of the ectoderm (see Chapter 3). It is induced to form early in the third week (about 18 days) by the developing notochord and the associated paraxial mesoderm.

The neural plate develops a longitudinal **neural groove** which has **neural folds** on each side (Fig. 17–1A). By the end of the third week, the neural folds have begun to fuse in the median plane to form the **neural tube** (see Fig. 17–1B).

The neural tube is the primordium (beginning) of the brain and spinal cord. The region where closure of the neural tube initially occurs corresponds to the future junction of the brain and spinal cord (see Fig. 17–4C). At first, the neural tube has open ends called the rostral and caudal neuropores (see Figs. 17–1B and 17–2A and C). The **rostral neuropore** closes on or before day 26 and the **caudal neuropore** closes before the end of the fourth week.

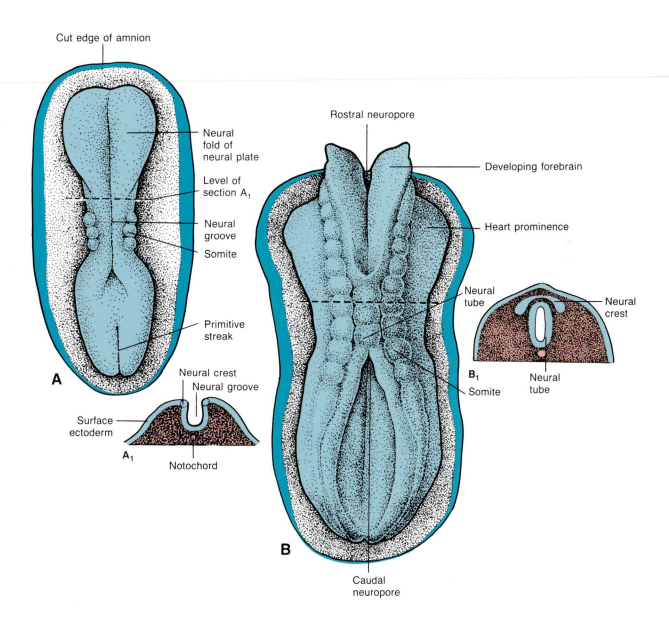

Figure 17–1 Drawing of embryos during the fourth week, illustrating early development of the central nervous system. *A*, dorsal view at 20 days; the amnion has been removed. The transverse section (*A₁*) illustrates the neural groove and neural folds. Note that as the neural folds fuse, some ectodermal cells lying along the crest of each neural fold form a mass known as the neural crest. *B*, dorsal view at 22 days. The neural folds have fused near the middle of the embryo to form the neural tube. The transverse section (*B₁*) illustrates the neural crest and neural tube. The neural tube is open at its rostral and caudal ends, where it communicates with the amniotic cavity through the rostral and caudal neuropores. Note that the neural folds at the rostral end have begun to thicken and form the brain.

As the neural tube forms and separates from the surface ectoderm (see Fig. 17–1A and B), cells from the neural folds aggregate to form a **neural crest** between the neural tube and the surface ectoderm. The *spinal ganglia* (dorsal root ganglia) of spinal nerves are derived from cells in the neural crest (see Figs. 17–1B₁ and 17–2B), as are comparable ganglia on the cranial nerves and autonomic ganglia, and the secretory cells of the medulla of the suprarenal gland (adrenal gland).

CENTRAL NERVOUS SYSTEM

Development of the Spinal Cord

The neural tube consists of three cellular layers (Fig. 17–3A). Nearest to the lumen is a thin **ventricular zone** (ependymal layer). External to this layer is the thick **intermediate zone** (mantle layer), and on the outside (see Fig. 17–2A) is the **marginal zone** (marginal layer).

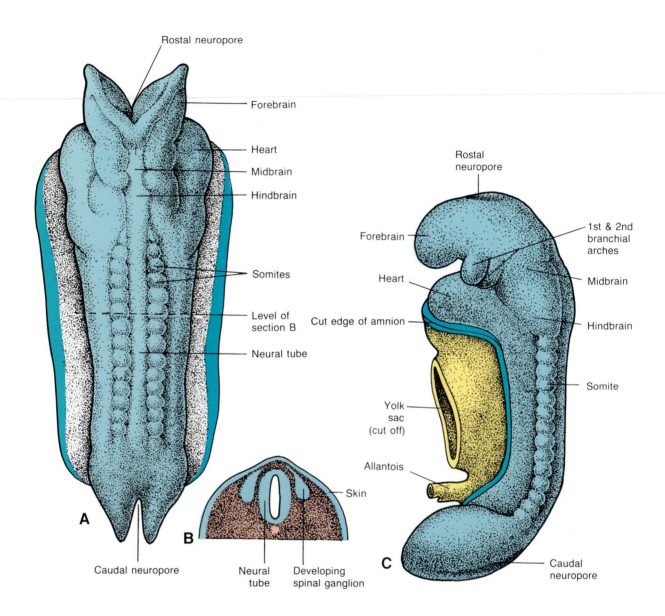

Figure 17–2 *A*, dorsal view of an embryo at 23 days. Note that the hindbrain and midbrain vesicles have formed and that the neural tube is much longer. The transverse section (*B*) illustrates spinal ganglia formed from the neural crest (see Fig. 17–1B₁) and the neural tube (future spinal cord). *C*, lateral view at 24 days. The rostral and caudal neuropores are still open. The rostral neuropore closes on day 25 or 26 and the caudal neuropore closes about two days later. Failure of these openings to close results in severe neural tube defects, such as meroanencephaly (anencephaly) and spina bifida with myeloschisis (see Figs. 17–5D and 17–6A).

Cells in the ventricular zone divide and produce two types of daughter cell: **neuroblasts** (future nerve cells) and **glioblasts** (future supporting cells called neuroglial cells). Both cell types complete their differentiation in the intermediate zone of the neural tube.

Laterally, on each side, there are two accumulations, or masses, of cells in the walls of the neural tube (developing spinal cord) that are separated by a shallow groove called the **sulcus limitans** (see Fig. 17–3A). The mass of cells dorsal to this groove is called the **alar plate** (lamina). The neurons that develop from neuroblasts in the alar plates are predominantly afferent or sensory. The mass of cells ventral to the sulcus limitans is known as the **basal plate** (lamina) and the neurons that develop from neuroblasts in this area are predominantly efferent or motor.

Cells in the alar plates give rise to the *dorsal*, or *posterior*, *horn of gray matter* (see Fig. 17–3C). In the thoracic and superior lumbar regions, a *lateral horn of gray matter* also develops. The ventral part of this horn, occupying the basal plate, is efferent. The basal plate gives rise to the *ventral*, or *anterior*, *horn of gray matter*. The neurons that develop from neuroblasts in the basal plate supply the skeletal muscle derived from the somites (see Chapter 15).

The enlarging ventral horns of gray matter bulge ventrally, creating the *ventral median fissure* (see Fig. 17–3C). The dorsal horns of gray matter approach each other, creating the *dorsal median septum* and obliterating the dorsal half of the lumen of the neural tube (see Fig. 17–3C). This creates the *central canal* of the spinal cord.

Length of the Spinal Cord.   For the first 12 weeks, the spinal cord is coextensive with the vertebral column so that the nerve roots pass directly into the intervertebral foramina. However, during later prenatal and postnatal development, growth of the vertebral column is greater than the spinal cord, owing to different growth rates and the degeneration of the caudal end of the spinal cord.

Because the cranial end of the spinal cord is attached to the brain, its caudal end progressively ascends in the vertebral canal. The *conus medullaris*, the tapered end of the spinal cord, is at the level of the third lumbar vertebra in newborn infants. The dura mater and arachnoid mater (layers of the meninges), however, still extend to the middle of the sacral canal (vertebral canal of the sacrum).

The membranes around the spinal cord, called *meninges*, contain a pool of **cerebrospinal fluid** (CSF) which can be tapped for diagnostic purposes. In the adult the spinal cord usually extends to the level of the first lumbar vertebra. Hence, when one is performing *spinal lumbar punctures* to obtain CSF, the needle is usually inserted between the vertebral arches of the third and fourth lumbar vertebrae to avoid damage to the spinal cord.

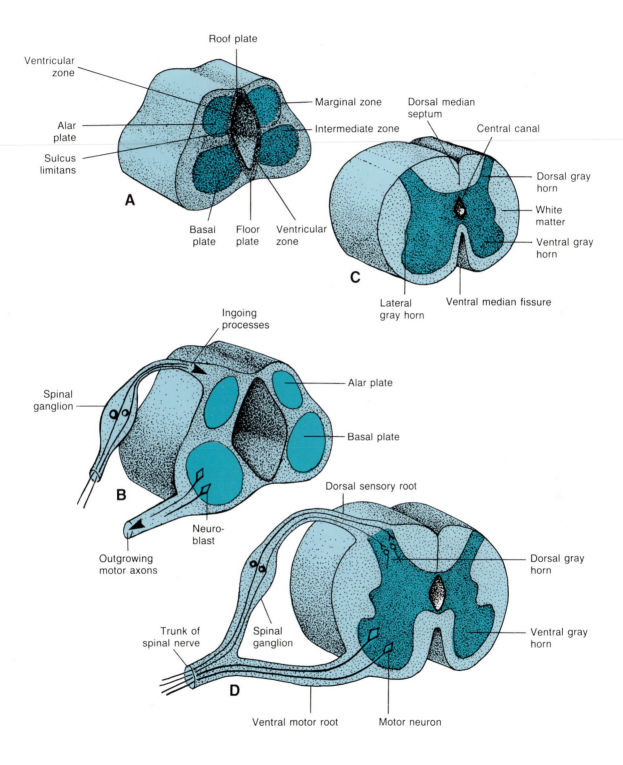

Figure 17–3 Drawings illustrating various stages in the development of the spinal cord and a spinal nerve. Note the formation of the dorsal and ventral gray horns from the alar and basal plates, respectively. *A*, six weeks. *B*, seven weeks. *C*, eight weeks. *D*, nine weeks. In *C* and *D*, observe the motor axons growing from cells in the ventral gray horn and the central and peripheral fibers growing from cells in the spinal ganglion. Note that the nerve fibers of the ventral motor root and the dorsal sensory root join to form the trunk of a spinal nerve.

TABLE 17–1   Development of the Brain from the Embryonic Brain Vesicles

Primary Brain Vesicles	Secondary Brain Vesicles	Region of Mature Brain
Hindbrain vesicle	Myelencephalon	Medulla
	Metencephalon	Pons and Cerebellum
Midbrain vesicle	Mesencephalon	Midbrain
Forebrain vesicle	Diencephalon	Thalamus, epithalamus, hypothalamus, and subthalamus
	Telencephalon	Cerebral hemispheres, consisting of the cortex and medullary center, the corpus striatum, and the olfactory system

The cavity of the hindbrain vesicle becomes the fourth ventricle; the cavity of the midbrain vesicle becomes the cerebral aqueduct, and the cavity of the forebrain vesicle becomes the lateral and third ventricles.

Development of the Brain

Even before the neural tube forms, the neural plate is expanded rostrally where the brain will develop (see Figs. 17–1B and 17–2). As the neural tube forms and the rostral neuropore closes, the thickened neural folds fuse to form three **primary brain vesicles**: the **forebrain** (prosencephalon), **midbrain** (mesencephalon), and **hindbrain** (rhombencephalon) (see Fig. 17–2). In Greek the brain is called *enkephalos*. The adult derivatives of these embryonic brain vesicles are shown in Table 17–1.

The development of the head fold in the fourth week (see Chapter 4) produces a **cervical flexure** in the neural tube near the junction of the hindbrain and the future spinal cord (Fig. 17–4A). As the brain vesicles enlarge, two other flexures form (see Fig. 17–4A to C): the **midbrain flexure** is convex dorsally in the midbrain region and the **pontine flexure** is convex ventrally in the hindbrain region (see Fig. 17–4B and C).

The Forebrain.   As the brain flexures form, the forebrain develops rapidly. During the fifth week it develops diverticula (outgrowths) called **optic vesicles** (see Figs. 17–4B and 18–1B) that will develop into the *eyes*, and **cerebral vesicles** that will become *cerebral hemispheres* (see Fig. 17–4C). The caudal part of the forebrain becomes the **diencephalon** (see Fig. 17–4D).

The cerebral vesicles enlarge rapidly, expanding in all directions until they cover the diencephalon and part of the brain stem (see Fig. 17–4E). In the floor and lateral wall of each vesicle, a thickening of nerve cells develops that will become the **corpus striatum** (see Fig. 17–4D), from which the *basal ganglia* will develop. Fibers from the developing cerebral hemispheres pass through the corpus striatum on their way to the brain stem and spinal cord, dividing the corpus striatum into two parts, the *caudate nucleus* and the *lentiform nucleus*. These fibers form the **internal capsule**.

Thickenings appear in the lateral walls of the diencephalon which will become the **thalamus**. The diencephalon also participates in the formation of the **pituitary gland** (hypophysis cerebri). The posterior lobe of the pituitary

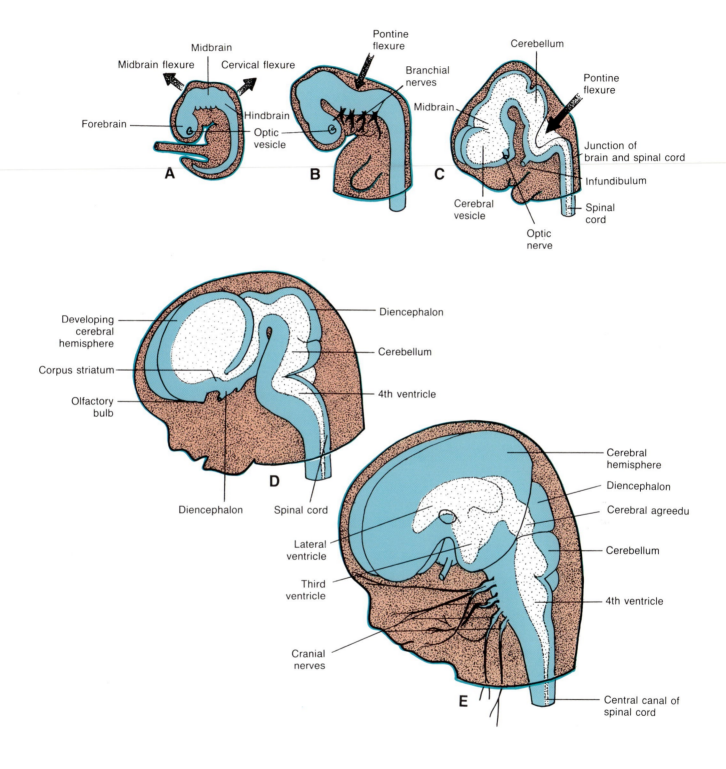

Figure 17–4 Drawings illustrating various stages in the development of the brain and the ventricular system. *A,* 28 days; *B,* 35 days; *C,* 56 days; *D,* 10 weeks; and *E,* 14 weeks. Note how the brain flexures affect the shape of the brain, enabling it to be accommodated in the head. Observe that as the cerebral hemispheres expand, they gradually cover the diencephalon and midbrain. Note how the nerves of the branchial arches, shown in *B,* become the cranial nerves, shown in *E.*

gland develops from a downgrowth from the diencephalon known as the *infundibulum* (see Fig. 17-4C). The anterior lobe of the pituitary gland develops from an evagination (upgrowth) of the *stomodeum* (primitive mouth cavity).

The Midbrain. The midbrain vesicle undergoes little change in becoming the adult midbrain, except for considerable thickenings of its walls (see Fig. 17-4C to E). It is the growth of large nerve fiber tracts through it that thickens its walls and reduces its lumen, which becomes the *cerebral aqueduct* (see Fig. 17-4E). The corticopontine and corticospinal fibers (fibers from the cerebral cortex going to the pons and spinal cord, respectively) are grouped on each side of the ventral surface of the midbrain, where they form the *crus cerebri* (cerebral peduncle).

Neuroblasts in the basal plates of the midbrain form the nuclei of two motor cranial nerves, the oculomotor and trochlear nerves (CN III and IV, respectively). The origin of cells in the red nucleus, substantia nigra, and reticular nuclei is uncertain. They appear to arise from the basal plates, but they may differentiate from cells that migrate from the alar plates.

The Hindbrain. The hindbrain divides into the myelencephalon and the metencephalon (see Table 17-1). The pontine flexure demarcates the division between these two parts (see Fig. 17-4B). Owing to the pontine flexure, the alar and basal plates in most parts of the hindbrain spread out like the opening of a book. As a result, these plates lie dorsolaterally and ventromedially, respectively.

The Myelencephalon. The caudal part of the myelencephalon becomes the closed part of the *medulla oblongata*. It resembles the spinal cord both developmentally and structurally. Neuroblasts from the alar plates form the *gracile nuclei* medially and the *cuneate nuclei* laterally. The *pyramids* of the medulla are composed of corticospinal fibers.

The rostral part of the myelencephalon becomes the "open" part of the medulla. Owing to the pontine flexure, this part of the medulla is wide and rather flat. The cells of *the basal plates form the motor nuclei of cranial nerves IX, X, XI, and XII* which lie in the floor of the medulla, medial to the sulcus limitans. The cells of *the alar plates form the sensory nuclei of cranial nerves V, VIII, IX, and X.* Other cells of the alar plates migrate ventromedially to form the *olivary nuclei*.

The Metencephalon. The ventral part of the walls of the metencephalon forms the *pons*. Cells in *the basal plates form the motor nuclei of cranial nerves V, VI, and VIII*, whereas cells in the ventromedial part of *the alar plates form the main sensory nucleus of cranial nerve V, a sensory nucleus of cranial nerve VII, and the vestibular and cochlear nuclei of cranial nerve VIII*. Cells from the alar plates also form the *pontine nuclei*.

The dorsal part of the walls of the metencephalon give rise to the mass of gray matter known as the *cerebellum*. The alar plates enlarge, project over the roof of the metencephalon, and fuse in the median plane to form the primordium of the cerebellum. At 12 weeks, the *vermis* and *cerebellar hemispheres* are recognizable. Some cells from the alar plates give rise to the *dendate nucleus* and other smaller cerebellar nuclei. The *superior cerebellar peduncles* consist mainly of fibers passing from the cerebellar nuclei to the midbrain.

Malformations of the Central Nervous System

Failure of the halves of the vertebral arch of one or more vertebrae to develop normally and fuse in the median plane results in a vertebral defect known as **spina bifida occulta** (Fig. 17–5A). If the meninges (membranes covering the spinal cord) project through the defect, they form a cystic swelling of the skin of the back that contains *cerebrospinal fluid*. This type of **spina bifida cystica** is known as **spina bifida with meningocele** (see Fig. 17–5B). The nervous system is usually normal.

Often the spinal cord and/or *cauda equina* protrudes into the membranous sac, forming a malformation known as **spina bifida with myelomeningocele** (see Fig. 17–5C). Neurologic deficits in the lower limbs and urinary bladder are common. Myelomeningoceles (also called meningomyeloceles) usually occur in the cervical and/or lumbar regions.

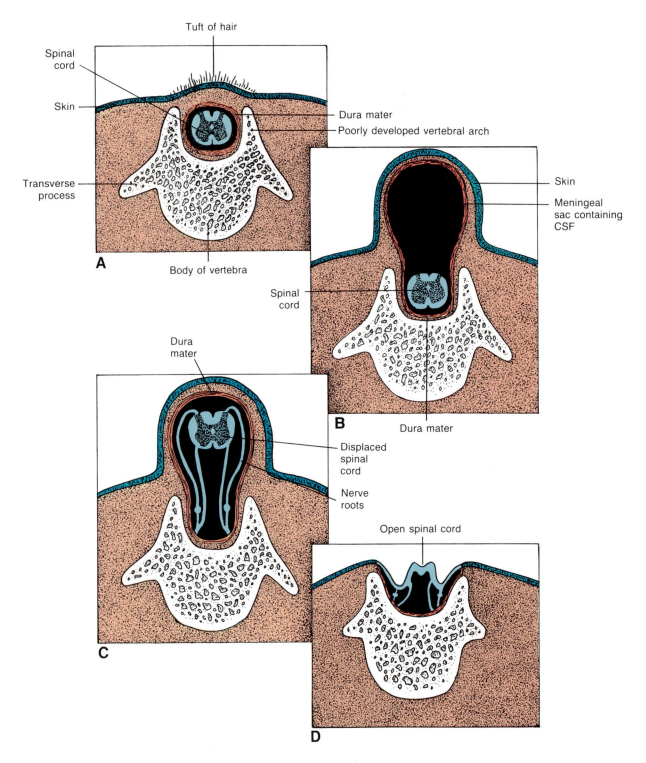

Figure 17–5 Schematic drawings illustrating the various types of spina bifida. *A,* spina bifida occulta, the most simple form, resulting from the failure of the halves of the vertebral arch to grow and fuse with each other. *B,* spina bifida with meningocele. When the arches of more than one vertebra are defective, the meninges bulge through the vertebral defects, forming a skin-covered meningeal sac. *C,* spina bifida with meningomyelocele. In this case, the spinal cord and its nerves have entered the meningeal sac which is covered by a thin, transparent membrane. Neurologic symptoms are often present, e.g., paralysis of the lower limbs. *D,* spina bifida with myeloschisis. Failure of the neural groove to close during formation of the neural tube (see Fig. 17–1A and B) results in exposure of the neural tissue of the spinal cord. In these cases, the defect in the vertebral arches is secondary to the defective neural tube formation. Myeloschisis is most common in the lumbosacral region, where it results from failure of the caudal neuropore to close.

The most severe type of spina bifida cystica is called **spina bifida with myeloschisis** or myelocele (see Fig. 17–5D). This malformation often *results from the failure of the caudal neuropore to close at the end of the fourth week.* Cerebrospinal fluid oozes from the central canal of the spinal cord over the raw nervous tissue. Owing to failure of development of the caudal part of the spinal cord and the spinal nerves, the lower limbs and pelvic organs are paralyzed.

Spina bifida cystica is sometimes associated with **meroanencephaly** (absence of the forebrain and midbrain). This *lethal malformation* of the brain, often inappropriately referred to as **anencephaly** (absence of the brain), *results from failure of closure of the rostral neuropore* during the fourth week. The cerebral hemispheres are absent and often the diencephalon and most of the midbrain are also absent (Fig. 17–6A). These infants are stillborn or die within a few hours or days after birth, usually from an infection of the exposed nervous tissue.

A defect in the formation of the cranium, called a **cranium bifidum**, is commonly associated with the herniation of the meninges or part of the brain through the defect. When the defect is small, usually only the meninges herniate, forming a meningial sac of cerebrospinal fluid called a **meningocele** (see Fig. 17–6B). If the defect in the cranium is large, part of the brain may herniate. This is known as a **meningoencephalocele**. These defects commonly occur in the occipital region.

In **microcephaly** (see Fig. 17–6C), the calvaria (cranial vault) is small. Microcephaly (small head) results from **microencephaly** (small brain). Normally the calvaria grows as the brain enlarges. Infants with these conditions are grossly mentally retarded. Microcephaly can result from exposure to large doses of radiation up to the sixteenth week of development, or from the effects of infectious agents (e.g., cytomegalovirus, herpes simplex virus, and *Toxoplasma gondii*).

In **hydrocephalus** there is an *accumulation of cerebrospinal fluid* in the ventricles of the brain (see Fig. 17–4E) and/or between the brain and dura mater. In the absence of surgical treatment, progressive enlargement of the ventricles results in atrophy of the cerebral cortex. In extreme cases, the head may be three times its normal size (see Fig. 17–6D).

Obstructive hydrocephalus (also known as internal hydrocephalus) usually results from narrowing or **stenosis of the cerebral aqueduct** (see Fig. 17–3E). This results in the enlargement of the lateral (first and second) and third ventricles. Obstruction of the foramina of the fourth ventricle results in the enlargement of all the ventricles. Hydrocephalus is often associated with spina bifida cystica and the **Arnold-Chiari malformation** (descent of the medulla oblongata and cerebellar vermis through the foramen magnum of the skull).

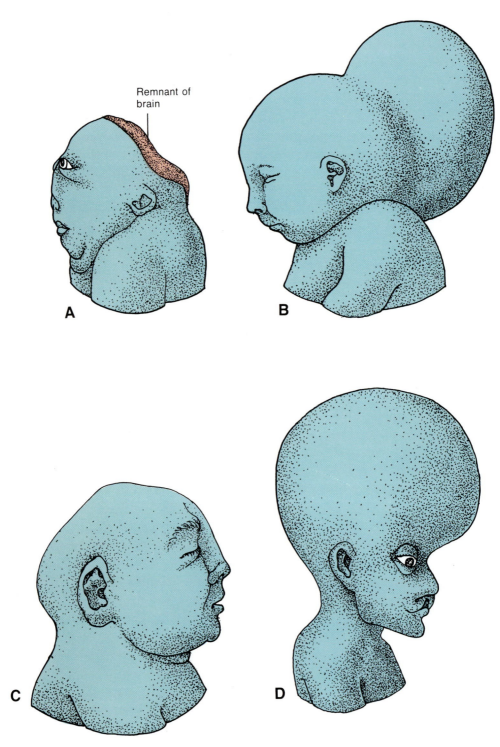

Figure 17-6   Drawings illustrating various types of malformation of the central nervous system. *A*, meroanencephaly (also known as anencephaly). Part of the brain is absent (G. *meros*, part). The cerebral hemispheres are absent and often much of the midbrain is deficient. The remnant of the brain appears as a reddish mass of nervous tissue that is exposed to the surface. *B*, cranium bifidum with meningocele or meningoencephalocele. The meninges or the meninges and part of the brain have bulged through the defect in the squamous part of the occipital bone. Meningocele, herniation of the meninges, is associated with small cranial defects. *C*, microcephaly (G. small head). The failure of the calvaria (cranial vault) to expand is secondary to failure of the brain to grow. This malformation is associated with severe mental retardation. *D*, hydrocephalus (G. water head) results from an excessive accumulation of cerebrospinal fluid in the ventricles of the brain. In most cases this malformation is associated with meningomyelocele, but hydrocephalus may result from stenosis of the cerebral aqueduct in the midbrain which often results from an intrauterine infection (e.g., by the rubella virus or cytomegalovirus).

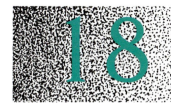

EYE AND EAR

EYE AND EAR

THE EYE

Development of the Eye and Optic Nerve

The eye is derived from three sources: **neuroectoderm** of the forebrain, **surface ectoderm** of the head, and **mesoderm** in the head (Fig. 18–1).

The primordia of neural parts of the eye are evident at the beginning of the fourth week, when **optic sulci** (optic grooves) develop in the neural folds at the cranial end of the embryo (see Fig. 18–1A).

Following closure of the rostral neuropore (see Fig. 17–4B), the optic sulci evaginate to form **optic vesicles** (see Fig. 18–1B). They project from the lateral walls of the forebrain in the region that later becomes the *diencephalon* (see Fig. 17–4D and Table 17–1). As the optic vesicles enlarge, their connections with the brain narrow to form hollow **optic stalks** (see Fig. 18–1C).

The optic vesicles approach the sides of the head and induce the surface ectoderm related to them to form thickenings called **lens placodes** (see Fig. 18–1B). As this occurs, the optic vesicles invaginate to form double-walled **optic cups** (see Fig. 18–1C). The invaginations also involve the ventral surfaces of the optic stalks where they form linear grooves called **optic fissures** (see Fig. 18–1C and E). The optic cups and fissures are filled with vascular mesenchyme from which the **hyaloid artery and vein** form. The hyaloid artery supplies the developing lens and the inner layer of the optic cup (see Fig. 18–1E and F).

Meanwhile, the lens placodes have sunk deep to the surface ectoderm where they form **lens pits**. As the lens pits deepen, they are gradually cut off from the surface ectoderm to form **lens vesicles** (see Fig. 18–1C and E). Their formation is also under the inductive influence of the optic vesicles.

The Retina. The retina is derived from the walls of the optic cup. Most of the *inner layer of the optic cup* thickens to form the *neural retina* (Fig. 18–2). The *outer layer of the optic cup* remains relatively thin and forms the *retinal pigment epithelium*. The original cavity of the optic cup is obliterated as the inner and outer layers fuse (see Fig. 18–2C), but this adherence is not firm. As a result, a blow to the eye may cause the separation of the neural retina from the retinal pigment epithelium, a condition known clinically as a *detached retina*. Anteriorly, the layers of the optic cup remain thin and form the nonvisual part of the retina.

The proximal parts of the hyaloid vessels form the *central artery and vein of the retina*. The distal parts of the hyaloid vessels disappear before birth (see Fig. 18–2C).

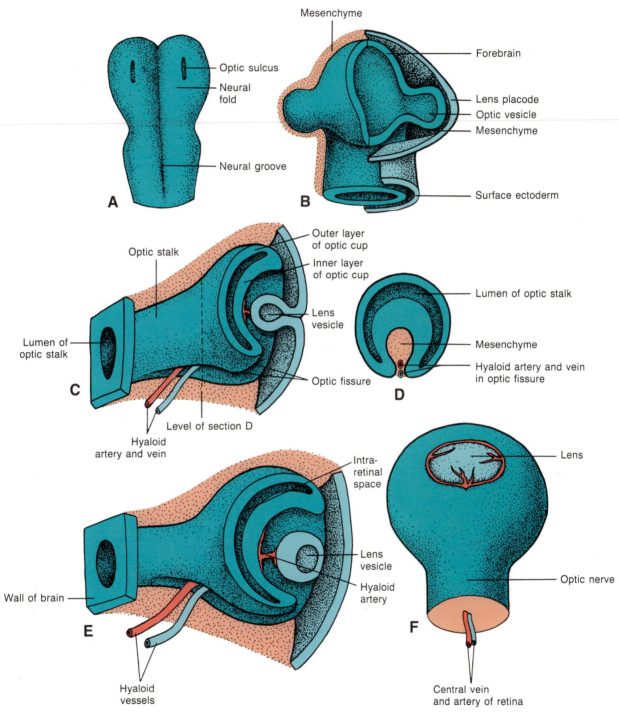

Figure 18–1 Drawings illustrating successive stages in the development of the eye. *A,* dorsal view of the cranial end of a 4-week embryo (about 22 days), showing the optic sulci (grooves). *B,* schematic drawing of the forebrain vesicle at the end of the fourth week, showing the optic vesicles that have grown laterally from the forebrain vesicle. Also observe the lens placode that has been induced to form from the surface ectoderm by the optic vesicle. *C,* drawing of the optic cup and the lens vesicle during the fifth week. Note the groove, known as the optic fissure, on the ventral surface of the optic cup and optic stalk. *D,* transverse section of the optic stalk, shown in *C,* illustrating the hyaloid vessels in the optic fissure and development of the optic nerve. *E,* drawing of the optic cup and lens vesicle during the sixth week. Note that the hyaloid artery runs in the optic fissure to supply the lens and the inner layer of the optic cup (future neural retina). *F,* ventral surface of the optic nerve and developing eye at the end of the seventh week, after closure of the optic fissure. At this stage the hyaloid artery supplies the lens, but this part of the artery degenerates in the fetal period (see Fig. 18–2C), leaving the lens avascular. Note that the proximal part of the hyaloid artery becomes the central artery of the retina.

The Optic Nerve. Each optic nerve is formed from the optic stalk and nerve fibers from the retina (see Fig. 18–1D and F). The axons of cells in the superficial layer of the neural retina grow proximally within the wall of the optic stalk to the brain. As this occurs, the cavity of the optic stalk is obliterated and the many nerve fibers from the retina form the *optic nerve* (see Figs. 18–1D and F and 18–2C). *Myelination of the optic nerves* begins late in the fetal period and is completed by the tenth week after birth.

The Ciliary Body and Iris. The anterior portion, or rim, of the optic cup grows over most of the anterior part of the lens. There it forms the epithelium of the ciliary body and iris (see Fig. 18–2B), as well as the *dilator and sphincter pupillae muscles* of the iris. The ciliary muscle and connective tissue in the ciliary body and iris are derived from the mesenchyme located around the rim of the optic cup.

The Lens. The lens is derived from the surface ectoderm (see Fig. 18–1B and C). The anterior wall of the lens vesicle remains thin and becomes the *anterior lens epithelium* (see Fig. 18–2B). The posterior wall of the lens vesicle thickens greatly, obliterating the lumen of the lens vesicle. The elongated cells of the posterior wall lose their nuclei and differentiate into *primary lens fibers.* Subsequently, *secondary lens fibers* are formed from epithelial cells at the equatorial zone of the lens (see Fig. 18–2B). This process continues during adult life.

The hyaloid artery supplies the embryonic and fetal lens (see Figs. 18–1E and 18–2), but the distal portion of this vessel disappears before birth. As a result, the lens is avascular and depends on diffusion from the aqueous humor and the vitreous body for its nutrition.

The Choroid, Sclera, and Cornea. The optic cup and optic stalk are surrounded by mesenchyme which is continuous with that surrounding the brain. This embryonic connective tissue differentiates into an inner layer that is continuous with the *pia and arachnoid layers of meninges* that cover the brain. This inner layer also forms the highly vascular *choroid* of the eye (see Fig. 18–2B). The outer layer of connective tissue is continuous with the dural sheath of the optic nerve and dura mater of the brain. This outer layer also forms the *sclera* of the eye and the *substantia propria of the cornea* (see Fig. 18–2B). Anteriorly, the *cornea* is covered with stratified squamous nonkeratinizing epithelium. This *anterior epithelium of the cornea* is derived from the **surface ectoderm** (see Fig. 18–2).

The Aqueous Chambers. The *anterior chamber* arises from a cavity that develops in the mesenchyme located between the developing iris and cornea (see Fig. 18–2B). The *posterior chamber* develops from a cavity that develops in the mesenchyme that lies posterior to the developing iris and anterior to the developing lens. The future pupil is initially covered by a layer of connective tissue called the **pupillary membrane** (see Fig. 18–2A). When this membrane disappears, usually by the twentieth week, the pupil forms and the anterior and posterior chambers communicate.

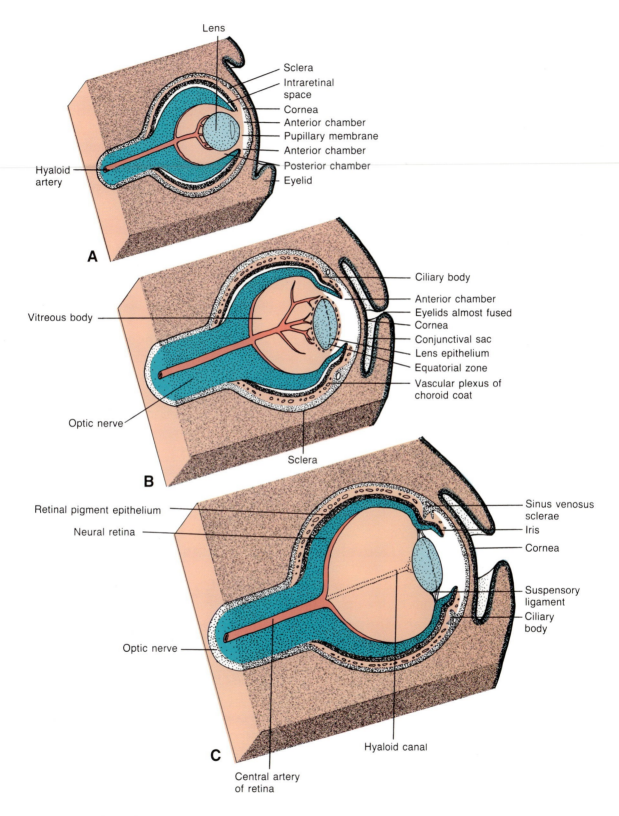

Lens

Sclera

Intraretinal space

Cornea

Anterior chamber

Pupillary membrane

Anterior chamber

Posterior chamber

Eyelid

Hyaloid artery

A

Ciliary body

Anterior chamber

Eyelids almost fused

Cornea

Conjunctival sac

Lens epithelium

Equatorial zone

Vascular plexus of choroid coat

Vitreous body

Optic nerve

Sclera

B

Retinal pigment epithelium

Neural retina

Sinus venosus sclerae

Iris

Cornea

Suspensory ligament

Ciliary body

Optic nerve

Hyaloid canal

Central artery of retina

C

Figure 18-2 Drawings of sagittal sections illustrating further stages in the development of the eye. *A*, 6 weeks; *B*, 20 weeks; and *C*, newborn. Note that the inner layer of the optic cup thickens to form the neural retina, whereas the outer layer remains relatively thin and forms the retinal pigmented epithelium. Also note that the cavity of the optic cup is obliterated by the fusion of these two layers. Observe that the anterior part of the optic cup grows partly over the lens to form the epithelium of the ciliary body and iris. Note that the cavity of the lens disappears as cells in its posterior wall elongate to form primary lens fibers.

The Vitreous Body.   This gelatinous mass is derived from the mesenchyme that enters the optic cup as it forms (see Figs. 18–1C and 18–2B). Some *vitreous humor*, the fluid component of the vitreous body, may be derived from the inner wall of the optic cup, particularly from the part that forms the epithelium of the ciliary body.

The Eyelids.   These accessory eye structures *develop from folds of the surface ectoderm* that form superior and inferior to the developing cornea (see Fig. 18–2A and B). The mesenchyme in the developing eyelids forms their connective tissue and the *tarsal plates*. The eyelids grow toward each other and adhere during the eighth week. They remain closed until about the twenty-sixth week.

Congenital Malformations of the Eye

Most common malformations of the eye are related to *defects of closure of the optic fissure* (see Fig. 18–1C to F). In **congenital coloboma**, the defect may involve the iris only, forming a split-like defect called a **coloboma of the iris**, or it may extend posteriorly into the ciliary body and retina forming a **coloboma of the retina.**

The developing lenses may be adversely affected by the *rubella virus* (German measles), causing them to become opaque. This severe condition is known as **congenital cataract**; it results in *blindness*.

Microphthalmos (small eye) is usually associated with other ocular abnormalities. This malformation commonly results from infectious agents (rubella virus, cytomegalovirus, and *Toxoplasma gondii*), but it is also associated with numerical chromosomal abnormalities (e.g., trisomy 13; see Chapter 7).

THE EAR

Development of the Ear

The development of the ear will be described in relation to its anatomical divisions and in the order that these divisions develop.

The Internal Ear.   The primordium of the internal ear is first indicated early in the fourth week by a thickening of the surface ectoderm which is called the **otic placode** (see Fig. 18–3B), that appears on each side of the hindbrain. This placode invaginates to form an **otic pit** (see Fig. 18–3B), the edges of which soon come together to form an **otic vesicle** or otocyst (see Fig. 18–3E). The otic vesicle soon loses its connection with the surface ectoderm (see Fig. 18–3D and E). A tubular diverticulum arises from the otic vesicle that will become the *endolymphatic duct and sac* (see Fig. 18–3F to H).

The otic vesicle soon becomes constricted near its middle to form a dorsal *utricular portion* and a ventral *saccular portion* (see Fig. 18–3F). The *semicircular ducts* arise from flattened outgrowths from the utricular portion of the otic vesicle (see Fig. 18–3G). The *cochlear duct* grows out from the saccular portion and spirals to form the *cochlea* (see Fig. 18–3H). A special neuroreceptor concerned with hearing, the *spiral organ* (of Corti), differentiates in the wall of the cochlea.

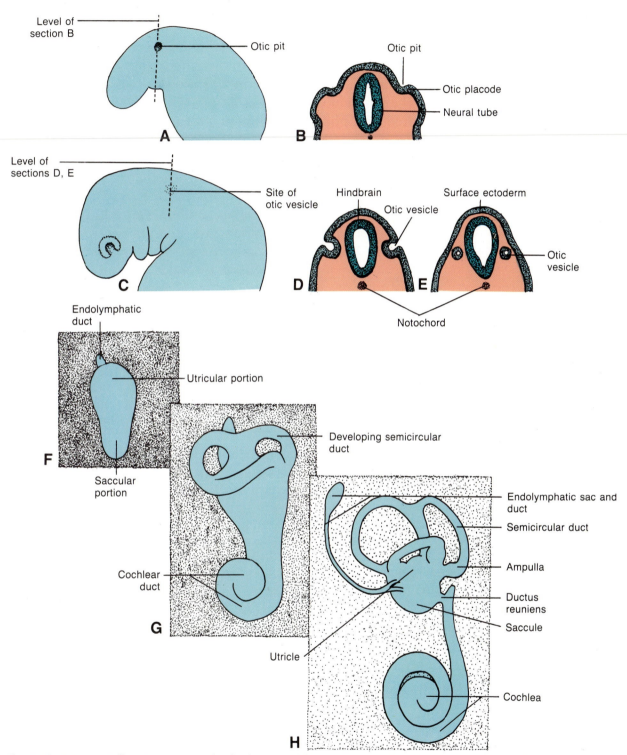

Figure 18–3 Drawings illustrating stages in the development of the membranous labyrinth of the internal ear. *A*, lateral view of the cranial end of a 4-week embryo (about 24 days), showing the location of the otic pit. *B*, schematic transverse section of the embryo shown in *A*. Note that the otic placode has receded beneath the surface ectoderm and lies in the floor of the otic pit. *C*, lateral view of the cranial region of a 4-week embryo (about 28 days), showing the location of the otic vesicle deep to the surface ectoderm. *D* and *E*, schematic transverse sections of the embryo shown in *C*. Observe how the otic pit sinks in further and is cut off from the surface ectoderm to form the otic vesicle. *F*, the otic vesicle shortly after its formation, showing the diverticulum of its dorsal wall that forms the primordium of the endolymphatic duct and sac. Note that the otic vesicle is constricted near its middle, forming utricular and saccular portions. *G*, the developing membranous labyrinth at 7 weeks showing the semicircular ducts that have developed as outgrowths from the utricular region of the otic vesicle. *H*, the membranous labyrinth at 8 weeks. Note that the cochlear duct has grown in the form of a spiral to form the cochlea. The spiral organ (of Corti) differentiates in its wall.

The derivatives of the otic vesicle constitute the *membranous labyrinth* that contains *endolymph*. The mesenchyme surrounding the developing membranous labyrinth chondrifies to form a cartilaginous **otic capsule**, which later ossifies to form the *bony labyrinth* that is located in the petrous part of the *temporal bone*. The mesenchyme between the bony and membranous labyrinths undergoes cavitation to form the *perilymphatic space* that contains *perilymph*.

The Middle Ear.   The tympanic cavity (see Fig. 18–4D) is derived from an extension of the elongated **first pharyngeal pouch**, an endodermal diverticulum of the primitive pharynx (see Chapter 9). This pouch expands to form the **tubotympanic recess** (see Fig. 18–4B), which grows laterally and approaches the floor of the **first branchial groove** (see Fig. 18–4D). The flattened end of the tubotympanic recess, together with the associated mesoderm and the ectoderm of the first branchial groove, form the *tympanic membrane* (see Fig. 18–4F).

The distal expanded portion of the tubotympanic recess soon becomes the *tympanic cavity* (see Fig. 18–4D). As the tubotympanic recess expands, it envelops the *auditory ossicles* (middle ear bones), which develop by endochondral ossification of the dorsal ends of the *cartilages in the first and second branchial arches* (see Fig. 18–4B). The proximal part of the tubotympanic recess becomes restricted to form the *auditory tube* (see Fig. 18–4D and F). An extension of the tubotympanic recess later forms the *mastoid antrum*. Most *mastoid cells* develop after birth, producing bulges of the temporal bones known as *mastoid processes*.

The External Ear.   The auricle of the external ear develops from six mesenchymal swellings, called **auricular hillocks**, that develop around the dorsal ends of the first and second branchial grooves (see Fig. 18–4A). These hillocks fuse to form the *auricle* (see Fig. 18–4C and E).

The *external acoustic meatus* develops from the dorsal portion of the first branchial groove (see Fig. 18–4B). Until the twenty-eighth week, the medial end of this meatus is plugged with a mass of epithelial cells called the **meatal plug** (see Fig. 18–4D). It normally disappears before birth (see Fig. 18–4F).

Congenital Malformations of the Ear

Infectious agents may affect development of the internal and/or middle ear and cause **congenital deafness** (deaf-mutism). It is well established that the *rubella virus* may cause abnormal development of the *spiral organ* (of Corti). Similarly, *Treponema pallidum*, the microorganism that causes syphilis, can damage the developing spiral organ if it crosses the placental membrane and enters the embryo's blood during the seventh week, the critical period of internal ear development. In about one-third of the cases of congenital deafness, genetic factors are involved.

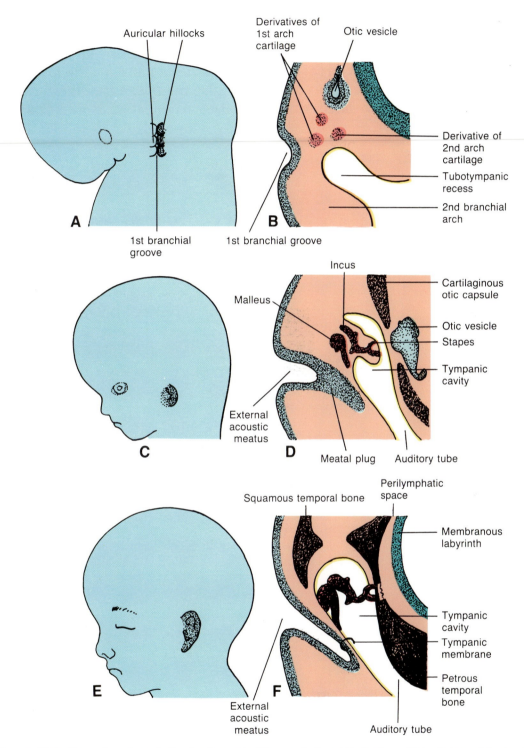

Figure 18–4 Diagram illustrating various stages in the development of the ear. *A, C,* and *E,* drawings of lateral views of the heads of 4- to 32-week embryos–fetuses, illustrating development of the auricle of the external ear from six swellings, called auricular hillocks. Note that they develop around the dorsal extremity of the first branchial groove. The hillocks fuse as the auricle forms. *B, D,* and *F,* schematic frontal sections of 4- to 8-week embryos, showing development of the external acoustic meatus, tympanic membrane, auditory ossicles, and tympanic cavity. Note that the tubotympanic recess develops from the first pharyngeal pouch and envelops the auditory ossicles. At the same time, the external acoustic meatus develops from the first branchial groove. The tubotympanic recess and external acoustic meatus meet as a film of mesoderm grows between them. The ectoderm of the external acoustic meatus, the endoderm of the tubotympanic recess, and the mesoderm between constitute the primordium of the tympanic membrane (eardrum). Note that the connection of the tubotympanic recess with the pharynx becomes the auditory tube (eustachian tube).

Abnormal fusion of the auricular hillocks can cause **malformed auricles**, as occurs when there is trisomy of the autosomes (e.g., trisomy 13 and trisomy 18; see Chapter 7). Infants with the **first arch syndrome** (see Chapter 7) also have malformed auricles, in addition to facial and other ear abnormalities.

Atresia of the external acoustic meatus results when the first branchial groove closes or the embryonic meatal plug persists. Again, these conditions are frequently associated with other *branchial arch anomalies* (see Chapter 9).

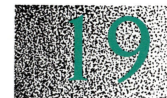

INTEGUMENTARY SYSTEM

INTEGUMENTARY SYSTEM

SKIN AND ITS APPENDAGES

The integumentary system consists of the skin and its appendages (e.g., hair, glands, and nails), and includes the mammary glands and teeth.

Development of the Skin

The *epidermis* is derived from the **ectoderm** which covers the surface of the embryo. The *dermis* is derived from the **mesoderm** underlying the surface ectoderm.

Initially, the **epidermis** consists of a single layer of ectodermal cells (Fig. 19–1A), but by the seventh week two layers of cells have formed: a superficial layer called the **periderm** and a deep layer called the **basal layer** (see Fig. 19–1B). Peridermal cells are continuously sloughed and are later mixed with hair and the secretions of the sebaceous glands to form a whitish substance called the **vernix caseosa** (see Fig. 19–1G). This greasy material protects the skin and probably makes it more waterproof.

The basal layer of the epidermis becomes the *germinal layer* which proliferates to form the stratified keratinizing epithelium known as the epidermis (see Fig. 19–1C and D). *Melanocytes*, the cells which produce the melanin that gives the skin its color, are derived from the **neural crest** (see Fig. 17–1B$_1$).

The *dermis* is formed from mesoderm which gives rise to the mesenchyme underlying the epidermis (see Fig. 19–1B). It is derived from two sources: the somatic mesoderm of the body wall and limbs, and the **dermatomes** (see Fig. 15–1A). Mesenchymal cells migrate from the somites and lateral mesoderm, bringing their innervation with them.

Development of Hairs

Hairs are formed from hair bulbs that develop from proliferations of the epidermis that grow into the dermis (see Fig. 19–1E). The deep end of each *hair bulb* is invaginated by mesenchyme that forms the *hair papilla* in which vessels and nerve endings develop (see Fig. 19–1F). Cells in the center of the hair bulb become keratinized to form a *hair shaft*, and its peripheral cells form the *epithelial root sheath*. The surrounding mesenchymal cells form the *dermal root sheath* and the *arrector pili muscle* (see Fig. 19–1G). This smooth muscle received its name because it makes the hair erect when it contracts.

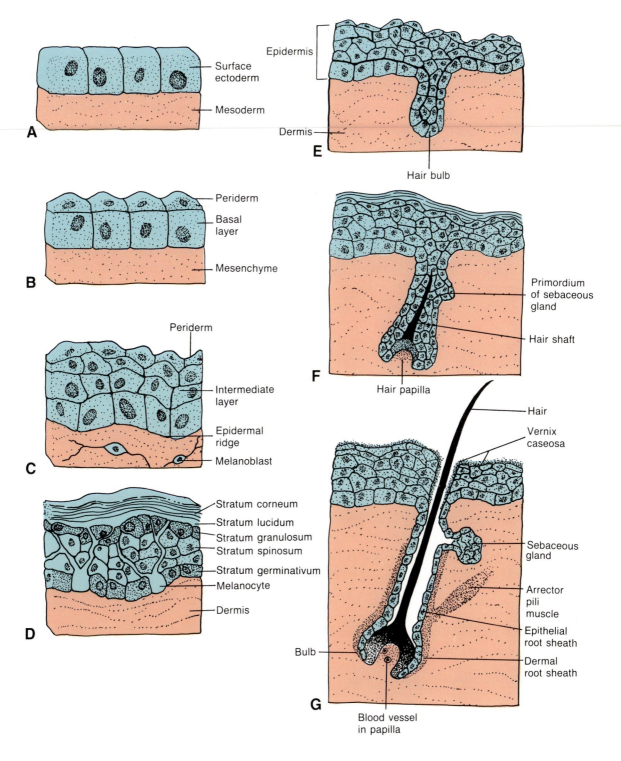

Figure 19–1 Drawings illustrating the development of skin and related structures. *A* to *D*, stages in the development of thick skin (4, 7, 11, and 36 weeks, respectively). Note that the skin is composed of two distinct parts, the epidermis and dermis, and that the epidermis is derived from the surface ectoderm and the dermis from the underlying mesoderm. *E* to *G*, stages in the development of a hair and a sebaceous gland (14, 16, and 18 weeks, respectively). The first hairs to appear, called lanugo hairs, are fine and difficult to see in young fetuses. These hairs are shed during the perinatal period and are replaced by coarser hairs.

The continuous proliferation of cells at the base of the hair shaft pushes the hair to the surface, where it protrudes through the epidermis (see Fig. 19–1G). The first hairs, called **lanugo hairs**, appear on the eyebrows and upper lip at the end of the twelfth week, but they are difficult to see. They cover the entire body by the twentieth week. These fine hairs are continuously produced and shed. Lanugo hairs are lost by the time of birth, or shortly thereafter, when they are replaced by coarser hairs.

Melanoblasts arise from the **neural crests** and invade the hair bulbs. Here they differentiate into *melanocytes* which produce melanin, which is deposited in the cells that form the hair shaft. In this way the hairs become colored.

Development of the Glands of the Skin

On the side of the hair follicle there are usually several sebaceous glands. Most *sebaceous glands* develop as outgrowths from the sides of hair follicles (see Fig. 19–1F and G) and discharge their secretion into the space around the hair. This secretion, called *sebum*, passes to the surface of the skin and forms the main component of vernix caseosa (see Fig. 19–1G). Some sebaceous glands develop as downgrowths of the epidermis into the dermis.

Sweat glands develop from the epidermis in a similar manner, except that the terminal part of each downgrowth coils to form the body of the gland. The central cells degenerate to form the lumen of the gland and the peripheral cells differentiate into secretory cells and contractile *myoepithelial cells*.

Development of the Nails

The first indications of developing nails are thickenings of the epidermis, called *nail fields*, which develop at the tips of the digits during the tenth week. The nail fields grow dorsally and proximally until they reach the normal position of the nails. As the nails develop they grow slowly towards the tip of the digits, which they usually reach before birth.

THE MAMMARY GLANDS

The mammary glands begin to form in the sixth week as downgrowths of the epidermis along the cranial parts of the **mammary ridges** (Fig. 19–2A and B). The glands develop by the sprouting of mammary buds (see Fig. 19–2C) which form numerous cords. These are slowly canalized to form *lactiferous ducts* (see Fig. 19–2E). At birth the rudimentary mammary glands are identical in both sexes.

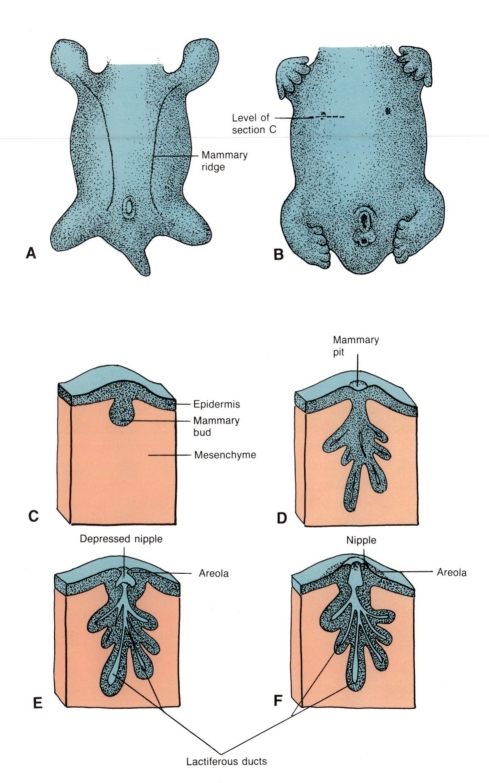

Figure 19-2 Drawings illustrating development of the mammary glands. *A* and *B*, ventral views of embryos at 4 and 6 weeks, respectively, showing the mammary ridges from which the mammary glands develop. *C* to *F*, transverse sections of developing mammary glands showing the epidermal cords that are canalized to form lactiferous ducts. *E*, at birth the rudimentary glands are identical in both sexes. *F*, during childhood the nipple usually elevates.

The nipples are depressed at birth, but normally become elevated during childhood (see Fig. 19–2F). Failure of this process to occur results in **inverted nipples.** At puberty the breasts in females normally enlarge owing to the growth of the mammary glands and the deposition of fat.

Fragments of the mammary ridges may persist and downgrowths from them may give rise to **supernumerary breasts** (*polymastia*) and **additional nipples** (*polythelia*). These breasts or nipples may develop anywhere along the original mammary ridges (see Fig. 19–2A).

THE TEETH

Two sets of natural teeth develop: the primary dentition or **deciduous teeth** and the secondary dentition or **permanent teeth.** *The teeth develop from ectoderm and mesoderm* (Fig. 19–3).

The first indication of tooth development occurs in the sixth week when U-shaped *thickenings of the oral ectoderm,* called **dental laminae,** develop in the maxilla and mandible (see Fig. 19–3A). At ten locations in each jaw, the dental lamina proliferates and produces downgrowths into the underlying mesenchyme called **tooth buds** (see Fig. 19–3B). The deep surface of each tooth bud is soon invaginated by mesenchyme which gives it a cap-like appearance (see Fig. 19–3C). Its ectodermal part is known as the **enamel organ** because it subsequently *produces enamel.* The invaginated part that is filled with mesenchyme called the **dental papilla.** It is the primordium of the *dental pulp.*

As the enamel organ grows, the developing tooth becomes bell-shaped (see Fig. 19–3D and E). Its external layer is called the *outer enamel epithelium* and its internal layer is called the *inner enamel epithelium.* The cells of the inner epithelium are called **ameloblasts.** Under their influence, the outer cells of the dental papilla differientiate into **odontoblasts.** The ameloblasts lay down *enamel* and the odontoblasts form *dentin.* The remaining cells of the dental papilla become the *dental pulp* which is invaded by vessels and nerves.

The vascular mesenchyme surrounding the developing tooth forms a **dental sac** (see Fig. 19–3E). It gives rise to *cementum* and the *periodontal ligament* which attaches the teeth to the *alveolar processes* (bony sockets). As the roots develop, the teeth erupt through the *gingiva* or gum (see Fig. 19–3G). The mandibular incisor teeth are the first to erupt, usually six to eight months after birth (see Fig. 19–3H).

Occasionally the incisor teeth have erupted at birth. These **natal teeth** are usually abnormally formed and have very little enamel and no roots.

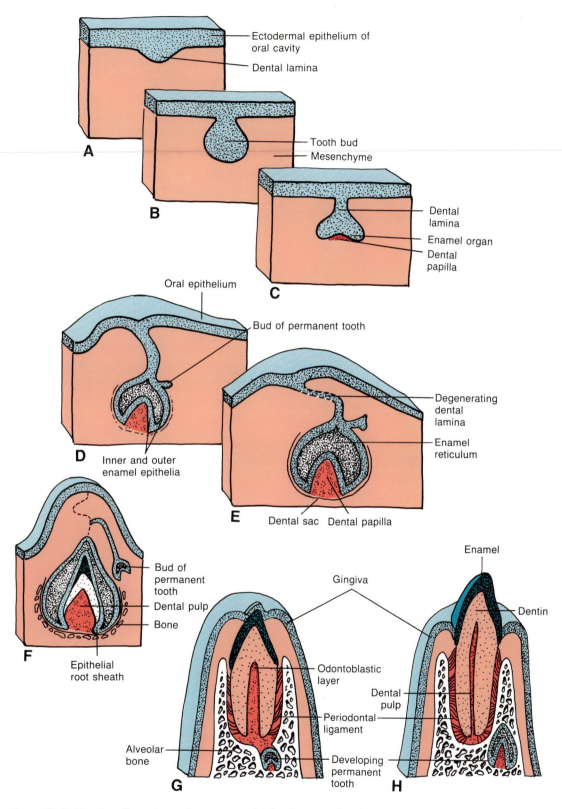

Figure 19–3   Drawings illustrating various stages in the development of teeth. *A,* 6 weeks; *B,* 7 weeks; *C,* 8 weeks; *D,* 10 weeks; *E,* 14 weeks; *F,* 28 weeks; *G,* 6 months after birth and *H,* 18 months after birth. Note that the ectodermal part of the tooth *(blue),* called the enamel organ, is molded over the mesodermal dental papilla *(red)* which becomes the dental pulp. Observe the early development of the primordium of a permanent tooth from the dental lamina of the deciduous tooth *(D to H).*

The buds of the permanent teeth begin to appear as early as the tenth week before birth (see Fig. 19–3D). On the lingual aspect of each developing deciduous tooth, a tooth bud for the permanent tooth arises from the dental lamina. Its development is the same as that of the deciduous teeth. The eruption of permanent teeth begins seven to eight years after birth.

Although **tooth abnormalities** are usually hereditary in nature, environmental agents such as the rubella virus, *Treponema pallidum* (syphilis), and high doses of radiation are known to cause abnormal development of the teeth.

Tetracyclines should not be administered to pregnant women or to children because these drugs adversely affect tooth development (*brownish-yellow discoloration* and **enamel hypoplasia**).